FEEL GOOD
LOOK YOUNGER

EDWIN LEE, M.D., F.A.C.E.

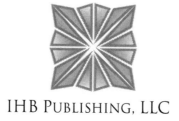

IHB Publishing, LLC

Your Life-Altering Guide to...

Feel Good Look Younger

Reversing Tiredness Through Hormonal Balance
(Second Edition)

Edwin Lee, M.D., F.A.C.E.

DrEdwinLee.com

Published in the United States of America by
IHB Publishing, LLC, Florida, USA

Library of Congress Cataloging-in-Publication Data
Feel Good Look Younger: Reversing Tiredness Through Hormonal Balance
Edwin Lee, M.D., F.A.C.E.
Library of Congress Control Number: 2013937028

ISBN: 978-0-9829193-4-7

Printed in the United States of America
Second Edition

DEDICATED TO MY WONDERFUL WIFE, SU-EUN,

WHO SUPPORTS ME BEYOND MY DREAMS;

TO MY SONS, CONNOR AND NATHAN,

WHO I PRAY WILL ALWAYS BE HEALTHY AND HAPPY;

AND TO MY PARENTS, STEWART AND YOUNG-JA,

WHO HAVE HELPED GUIDE MY JOURNEY IN LIFE.

"Dr. Edwin Lee has taken the elegant,

simplex approach to hormone balance by

making a complicated topic easy to understand.

His book is a masterful, scientific and artful representation

of how to effectively get back energy and vitality

in tired, chaotic, stressful times."

— Deanna Minich, Ph.D., F.A.C.N., C.N.S.
author of Chakra Foods for Optimum Health
and The Complete Handbook to Quantum Healing

ACKNOWLEDGEMENTS

I would like to thank Jim Huth for helping me achieve my dream. I have always wanted to write a book, and without his encouragement I would never have realized my dream. To bring this book to print, Jim spent countless hours and many all-nighters, all of which had me worrying about him developing adrenal fatigue and harming his health with his crazy work schedule! I am so grateful for his gift in writing. It has been a great experience working with Jim.

Without my wonderful staff I would be in trouble. I would like to thank: Jason Holland, my assistant, who is as passionate about health as I am and is always curious about how the body works; Susan Hyatt, for her remarkable medical and laboratory skills; Kari Savage, for her wonderful knowledge of nutritional supplements and her live blood analysis skills; and Debra Broom, for her punctuality and also her organizational skills.

In addition, I would like to thank Mike Potthast for developing the cover of the book in such a short time. He is an amazing artist and a great friend. Thanks, as well, to Susan Davis and Allison Kaylor for their excellent grammar checking skills.

I would also like to thank my brother, Richard Lee, for helping me obtain medical references, and my family for their unwavering moral support.

Of course, my patients have my most genuine gratitude as well. I sincerely thank my patients for allowing me to participate in their health care.

TABLE OF CONTENTS

FOREWORD

"You will benefit from his journey."
— Florence Comite, M.D.

When I first met Dr. Lee in 2010 at the Age Management Medicine conference, I was thrilled to meet a fellow endocrinologist focused on health. Treating the body as a whole and identifying potential for disease rather than treating symptoms is the future of medicine. Most people only go to a doctor when they are sick or suffer an injury, the presumption being, if you keep the doctor away, you too are good to go, healthy, fine. This may not be the case, however. You could have underlying issues like diabetes or high cholesterol—not necessarily disease announced in red, flashing lights like a heart attack or stroke, but problem children all the same. Advances in medicine allow us to detect alterations in your body's metabolism decades before most women and men are told by their doctor, "You are a diabetic." Wouldn't it be better to work in partnership with your doctor to reverse this path to debilitating diseases, or even prevent them altogether before they arise? This is how I see medicine, and Dr. Lee has a similar vision.

It was at that biannual Age Management Medicine conference when I quickly learned that Dr. Lee was what I call a "forward-thinking" endocrinologist, an early adopter of advancing technology, and more importantly, open to alternative interventions.   Endocrinologists are primed to see connections throughout the body. As a field, it's all about messengers and systemic communication. In fact, there's a large-scale study starting in Australia where investigators are recruiting men who are pre-diabetic. (They're hoping to get 1,500 participants.) Men who match the research criteria will either be given injections of testosterone or a placebo, the goal being to illuminate the relationship testosterone has with other physiological processes outside the realm of sexual function and reproductive health. There haven't been many formal studies to date that explore testosterone's effect on insulin sensitivity, and so investigations like this, however rare, give me hope. It's a sign of a change in how medical clinicians view the body—that we're beginning to see disorders and interventions, as not in a direct cause and effect relationship, but rather as multi-factorial processes that may produce various interactions throughout the body, with innumerable outcomes.

While trained to focus on interactions (which is good), the downside is that as a class of specialists, endocrinologists (in general) tend to be a conservative bunch, typically drawn to bench research. Many are used to seeing diabetics, for instance, with blood work that is alarming—a hemoglobin A1C of 7.5, or even as high as 12 (while national guidelines give a cutoff of 5.7 as a pre-diabetic, I like to see my patients hover around 5 or less); a fasting insulin of less than 5 (this number should be zero!)—yet little is done to help these patients. In fact, it is likely that newscaster Tim Russert had these unacceptable lab findings, likely out of the healthy range, when he died of a sudden heart attack at 58 in the prime of his life. Generally those like Russert may get a few words of guidance: You're okay. Just try to watch your weight, stop eating too many sweets, or lose a few pounds, get to the gym, reduce the stress in your life. While this advice is sound, it is also generic, without specific guidance that applies to the individual living his or her life; Dr. Lee and I would not stop there. We believe reference ranges are too lenient, already evident of disease that has been smoldering for years, and many doctors don't even test hormone biomarkers like cortisol, estrogen, progesterone, testosterone, DHEA, or thyroid tests such as T3, and T4.

Often under-appreciated and therefore overlooked, all of these are critically important to the body's functioning. Dr. Lee and I view hormonal optimization as a major contributor to keeping your health and a good quality of life as the years tick upward.

Aging happens at the cellular level long before it shows in the wrinkles on our skin and the need for a cane or walker. We need to build in health at the front end of life through optimization of hormones, metabolism, the immune system, while lowering inflammatory markers, among other factors. No matter if you are 17 or 77, we can live through each year without feeling older, and possibly even get healthier as we add candles to our birthday cakes. At the core of this process, in my view, is the relationship between your personal medical history, your genetic make-up, and your lifestyle. For instance, sleep is when many of our hormones are released, so if you are skipping out on those precious hours with your blanket and pillow, you may be more than just tired. You may also have decreased melatonin levels and elevated cortisol (stressor) hormone. Add to that a genetic predisposition for obesity and some extra weight around the middle, and you may have sleep apnea. Apnea would further disrupt your sleep and deprive your body of oxygen, ultimately increasing your risk of hypertension, diabetes, heart disease, and, yes, even early death. You see, it's all connected.

Your body is replete with cells that interact in complex ways, and Dr. Lee understands that for each person a highly individualized process is required to get all your systems working in concert. We both find it gratifying to see our patients' primary goal be healthy living and not just recovery or rehab. Tracking our patients' progress—providing them with the medical wisdom to interpret the personal knowledge and medical metrics they gather along this journey—is ever rewarding. Disease-centric models of medicine are dated. It is absolutely necessary that we flip our perspective to being prospective, focused on the standpoint of well being and sustaining health for life. We want to choose to live life to the fullest for as long as possible, not settling for the slide that's bound to happen when we do nothing until disease occurs. Proactively working to maintain our physiological peak is the direction in which I want medicine to go, and Dr. Lee shares this sentiment.

We're beginning to live in the age of electronic medical records and digital devices that collect information on your heartbeat, your sleep patterns, your paces per day, all aiding in self-quantification. As the baby boomers age, it will be imperative that we each take control of our own health and not rely solely on our annual visit with a primary care physician to bring up any concerns we may have or reoccurring symptoms we might be experiencing. Dr. Lee examines a wide array of hormones and biomarkers, and he delves into the specifics of lifestyle, and functionality as well as sleep, exercise, nutrition and interpersonal relationships. With his guidance, patients learn more about themselves and are better able to take care of their health outside the confines of a doctor's office or hospital. This kind of mindful living alongside the care of a compassionate and insightful physician, such as Dr. Lee, is the way of the future.

There are serious health issues arising in America and around the world. The economic cost of health has skyrocketed due to diseases such as diabetes mellitus, which, Centers for Disease Control and Prevention estimates show, will affect one in every three adults living in the United States by 2050 if current trends continue. How do we relieve the national burden as well as the personal weight of aging? Today's disorders of aging—like diabetes, as well as autoimmune diseases, cancers, cardiovascular disease, dementia, malnutrition, nutrient deficiency, adrenal fatigue, muscular disorders, arthritic joint diseases, and osteoporosis—are but a few of many frailties that affect the way people live every day. I use the term disorders of aging, as it is my belief that by owning your health, age may not be synonymous with disease. Our bodies may stay strong and able, allowing us to play, dance, run, teach, think and feel (all those good action verbs), until our cells grow tired and we slip into death gracefully without the agony of prolonged disability. It is important to learn from the past and begin preventing instead of "curing." Chronic disorders happen within the body, not to the body, unlike infections which generally strike from without, it is our failing bodies that allow for diseases to take hold.

Chronic conditions such as heart disease, which is the number one killer of Americans, are byproducts of many years of oxidative stress, inflammation, inadequate diets, improper or imprecise nutrition, high levels of stress, lack of exercise and poor sleep. What's more, many of these health problems go undetected. For example, Dr. Lee begins his chapter on hypothyroidism by saying at least ten percent of American adults are believed to have underactive thyroids. That estimate means nearly 30 million people are hypothyroid, which is more than the number of people with diabetes and cancer, combined. Thyroid disorders, among others, may not be immediately perceptible, but rather compound over time and really begin to drag you down. You feel sluggish. It gets harder to get out of bed. Exercise, even sex, seems to be an afterthought that is only geared toward "young" people. The truth is that everyone still has the opportunity, and a right, to feel their best. Sleep, sex, diet, exercise and overall happiness are crucial components of well-being; and yet, most medical schools fail to teach their students about their relevance in a meaningful way, or frankly, at all. Actually, it is my belief that understanding the importance of our health needs to start earlier in life, as autopsy reports have revealed blocked and diseased arteries in young children who are killed in car crashes and 18-year-olds who die in combat. If decisions about food, drink and lifestyle begin in childhood, our nation will feel the impact in overall health.

I have a private practice on the Upper East Side of New York where my aim is to help patients sustain a good quality of life at any age. After much back-and-forth with those in my office and my colleagues, I've settled on the name: precision—age management—medicine. Before New York and a brief two-year stop in California where I set up a center at Ojai Valley Inn & Spa to integrate complementary and alternative medicine interventions with conventional medicine, I taught at Yale University School of Medicine. During that time, I also founded Women's Health at Yale and did extensive clinical research on the hypothalamic-pituitary-gonadal axis. It was actually (beginning at the NIH in the 1980s) when I studied children who were experiencing precocious puberty—a phenomenon where surges of testosterone and estrogen occur much earlier than would be expected in "normal" teen development—that I realized how hormones might be harnessed to maintain health as we mature past our 20s and 30s. The proper understanding of how hormones work and customizing the use of bioidentical hormones for each individual is a huge part of healthy aging. When we are no longer ideally suited to contribute to the gene pool through reproduction, our body tells itself to start slowing down. We can interrupt those signals and tell our body that there is still much vitality to be had in life. In my practice, I'd estimate that I see twice as many men to women. As such, I've focused my recent attention in gaining a deeper understanding of andropause (the male equivalent to menopause), and I employ various treatment methods including injections of human chorionic gonadotropin (also known as HCG) and testosterone. Testosterone gets a lot of bad press; however, the truth is that it is essential to our well-being. Lean muscle mass, sugar metabolism, sexual function and overall energy are all affected by adequate hormone levels.

Dr. Lee's particular area of expertise is adrenal fatigue. He explores how suboptimal levels of cortisol, aldosterone and DHEA contribute to fatigue and a general feeling of slowing down. Of course, Dr. Lee doesn't stop there. Just measuring these three hormones wouldn't give us the full picture, and so his revised edition of this book goes on to explore an array of other biomarkers and lifestyle components. There is a new emphasis on leaky gut syndrome, which—despite the somewhat-silly, over-obvious name—affects countless people. It's not just about what you eat, but also how or if you absorb those nutrients, and many of us have problems with both. This second edition also underscores the importance of the role that your hormones play in keeping your DNA healthy. With age, the ends of our DNA—called telomeres—begin to fray and unwind like a piece of rope that's coming undone. By keeping your estrogen, progesterone, testosterone, and even growth hormone levels optimal, you can keep your telomeres intact longer.

As already mentioned, the way Dr. Lee and I understand medicine is that it's complex, as well as interrelated. The brain, heart, thyroid—no organ can be studied in isolation. We are all puzzles, and our make-up is still an enigma; we only understand a fraction of how our system relates. Your lab work and medical history will help to give you clues on where each piece should be placed, and then it's up to you to partner with your physician to change your lifestyle for the better.

It is tough to get some doctors to address, let alone listen to your individual needs based on personal and family history, genetics, and environment. This is for good reason, though unfortunate, due to the current challenges in our overloaded health care system. Many doctors are pressed for time or need to move on to the next patient out of the many more that are in their waiting rooms. Dr. Lee expounds on the belief that a doctor should be able to take more than a few minutes to gather the information necessary to treat a patient properly, and his actions align with his words. Since much of what medicine purports to do, diagnose or manage, occurs outside of the doctor's office, it is essential to prepare patients for the health strains of day-to-day life. Sure, better patient education can lead to better health outcomes, but a key element patients really want is from their doctor to be compassionate, to understand what is important to us as individuals. Compassion heals. Someone once told me, "People pay for your brain, but pray for your heart." Success on the path to well-being takes the help of someone who is not only dedicated to fixing the numbers that show up on lab reports, then also cares enough to help you improve at your own pace and in a way that makes the most sense for you.

I remember Dr. Lee conveying the significance of his first time attending the Age Management Medicine Conference in 2007. He was so inspired to go beyond what conventional medicine was providing patients that he began an entirely new practice the next year, in the midst of the recession, to focus on the importance of nutrition and hormonal optimization. Today, Dr. Lee's Institute for Hormonal Balance is thriving in Orlando, Florida.

Most of what doctors practice is what they learn in medical school and training. Not Dr. Lee. Following his decades of education to become an endocrinologist, Dr. Lee recognized that in order to give his patients the best care he thought possible, he needed to make a huge leap of faith into the future of medicine and bring his vision to life. You will benefit from his journey.

— Florence Comite, M.D.

INTRODUCTION

"All truth passes through three stages.
First, it is ridiculed. Second, it is violently opposed.
Third, it is accepted as being self-evident."
— Arthur Schopenhauer

Sometimes it takes decades before a medical standard will change. In the 1800s, a Hungarian physician noted that washing hands before assisting in the delivery of babies reduced the death rates of infants. You see, during those times, it was common practice for doctors to work on cadaveric bodies and then turn around to deliver babies— without washing their hands! At first, an idea such as hand washing was ridiculed. It was not until Louis Pasteur later confirmed the germ theory, and hand washing finally began its transition from ridicule to self-evident truth.

Today, there are many controversial areas of endocrinology causing similar discord. Because of this, there are physicians who still consider these sources of discord to be taboo—something that should be kept secret. In the following chapters, I will address the "endocrinology secrets" of: adrenal fatigue (which is not yet considered a medical condition), the use of growth hormone, the use of T3 therapy in hypothyroidism or underactive thyroid, the use of progesterone for anything other than pregnancy, the use of estrogen, the use of testosterone and the use of DHEA.

All of these topics are based on confirmed clinical studies or have been reported in medical literature; however, with the current explosion and availability of medical news, it is almost impossible for any one physician to keep up with all the studies that are being published daily. And as we all know, sometimes when the truth lies right in front of us, it can be the hardest thing to see.

In addition to the secretive areas of hormonal balance—the controversial topics of endocrinology that deal with the issue of tiredness—I will address chronic inflammation, leaky gut, delayed food sensitivity and the benefits of intravenous nutrition.

To better understand, let us begin at the time in most people's lives— around 20 to 25 years of age—when, as a young adult, most people seem to feel their overall best. It's also the time that most people tend to hit their athletic peaks. Then, during your 30s or 40s, things start slowing down... as dictated by your hormones. But it doesn't have to always be that way.

Due to the fact that there are so many hormones that decline with age, your optimal hormonal balance is re-achieved by reintroducing those deficient hormones. Take melatonin, for example. When melatonin starts declining, you begin having problems with sleep— slowly at first, then much more noticeably as time goes by. Then, when melatonin is brought back into balance, your sleep improves.

Another example is progesterone deficiency, which is very common around 35 to 40. A proper balance of progesterone helps you relax and will calm you down. Without it you're irritable and anxious—and women experience a heavier menstrual cycle. But it is not just for women as I've prescribed progesterone for men as well. They say it takes the edge off, makes them more relaxed and calm.

Although you can't be 20 or 25 again, you can feel and function much better than you would with anything less than your optimal balance of hormones—that is, once you open the door to the incredible potential of hormonal balance and optimization. And the reason most people finally walk through that door is simply that they are tired of being tired.

"I was tired of always being tired."

I decided on my 53rd Birthday that I was tired of always being tired, over-whelmed, anxious, irritable and unable to sleep—and I didn't want to feel that way anymore! I'd read about bioidentical hormone replacement, but the doctors I spoke with were not familiar with it. Then I saw a magazine article about Dr Lee and I made an appointment with his office immediately.

From the beginning, I felt very comfortable with Dr. Lee. I was impressed with his expertise and the fact that, unlike other doctors, he really listened to me! After testing he started me on progesterone right away. I had been lacking this hormone for many years due to a partial hysterectomy at 42, and I started feeling much better within months. I was less irritable, less anxious, had more energy and was finally sleeping well!

It was then that I started to notice some of the symptoms I had experienced in two of my daughters. So I brought them in to see Dr. Lee and, just as expected... low progesterone and low serotonin levels in both of them—even though they are only 18 and 21! Now, they are both on bioidentical progesterone and doing great. The 18-year-old is less anxious and less irritable, and the 21-year-old is less irritable, plus her menstrual cycle is finally regular.

I highly recommend Dr. Lee and am always referring family and friends of all ages to the Institute for Hormonal Balance. Dr. Lee has improved my quality of life and helped my daughters. I'm sure he will continue to do the same for us and others.

— Deborah Broom

The most common complaint I hear in my office is, "I'm tired," or, "I have no energy." In response, I usually ask each patient to rate their overall energy in the past month on a scale from one to ten. The most frequent number I get is three. Sometimes I even hear zero! Then, after beginning treatment, when their energy numbers inevitably climb toward ten, I still get excited every time. However, my work hasn't always been so personally rewarding.

When I was practicing traditional endocrinology, if optimizing a patient's thyroid status didn't really help, I'd routinely defer them to their primary care physician. That was tough for me to do because, in the back of my mind, I always knew that somehow I could be helping —finding the cause rather than treating the symptom! However, at that time, I just didn't know where to turn within the constructs of my traditional medical training.

It was during those years, also, that I was honored to be Team Endocrinologist for the Cleveland Indians. Working almost daily with those athletes to maximize their health and physical potential is what sparked the catalyst for my success today. I believe that my experiences with those professional athletes and their need to be "at the top of their game"—when combined with my drive to overcome everyday tiredness—provided me with a very unique opportunity.

So, I dedicated myself to determining exactly what would put all of my patients "at the top of their game," and at last, I began to truly understand how your body can heal itself when given the proper nutrients, lifestyle modification, proper detoxification and, of course, hormonal balance.

Then, when I started seeing extraordinary improvements in the health of my patients by balancing their hormones, improving their nutritional status and safely disengaging them from some of their prescription medications, I knew I was onto something very significant. I was already board certified in Internal Medicine, Endocrinology, Diabetes and Metabolism; however, soon after completing special courses in Regenerative and Functional Medicine, I was able to help even more people reverse tiredness!

Yet, today, there is a troubling paradigm in medicine. According to the World Health Organization, the US ranks 37th in health care, yet is 1st in health care expenditures—clearly indicative that our medical system is based not on wellness, but on illness. For example, we now have an untreated epidemic of obesity in our children. Consequently, we're most probably in a generation where our children will grow into adults who will require massive health care expenditures for treating their weight-related medical conditions and ultimately may even die before their parents.

Someday, and hopefully soon, insurance companies will begin rewarding physicians for improving wellness (which will raise our health care status from its lowly 37th ranking). For example: helping patients lose weight, quit smoking or reduce their consumption of prescription medications. Which reminds me of the stories of doctors from China long ago, during a time when village doctors would not receive their monthly income if someone in their village became sick. The lesson to be learned from those old stories is simply that we need to be more proactive and less reactive.

So, I left conventional endocrinology to devote myself and my practice full time to the more proactive approach of hormonal balance. Once I did that, I realized that my true calling—my passion—was to help educate my patients. For you see, in conventional medicine, a doctor is not rewarded for educating you, or for warning you on the dangers of prolonged use of certain medications, or even for recommending alternative ways for you to address your problems.

However, in my private practice, I'm able to take my time with each patient—60 minutes with each new patient and 30 minutes or more with all returning patients throughout the course of my day, every day. This is time I'm investing to educate my patients (and you, through this book), thereby providing the knowledge and power to live a better, healthier life—and not just saying, "Take two of these every day until the bottle is empty."

For the physician, it all comes down to two things: the importance in knowing that everyone's metabolism and biochemistry are unique, which means there is not just one pill or cure that works for everyone; and…

…that you cannot simply treat one part of the body without impacting other—sometimes seemingly unrelated—parts of the body.

Doctors who understand this, are almost always the doctors who know they need to teach their patients. Educating my patients is paramount to me. After all, where else can you get the medical information vital for achieving optimal health, if not from your trusted physician? Sure, there's an incredibly voluminous amount of information on the Internet, but how much do you trust that it's all good and current information?

Throughout this book, I will be providing what is nothing less than the best and most reliable information on how you may reverse tiredness and live a healthier life. However, even though the following chapters address the secrets of hormonal balance and optimization, you cannot really begin to benefit from those secrets until you absolutely understand that the single most important step toward regaining your energy, feeling good and looking younger is...

...reducing chronic inflammation.

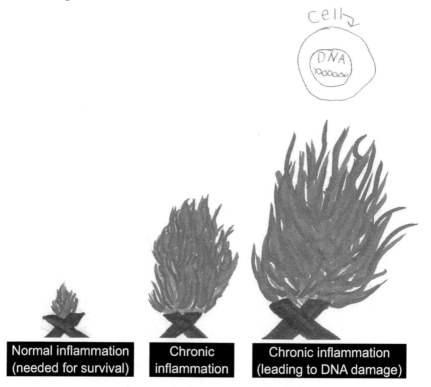

Thanks to some "commissioned" artwork from my sons, Connor and Nathan, the image of fire compares normal inflammation to chronic inflammation—which leads to DNA damage, which causes accelerated aging, chronic disease and cancer.

Artwork by Connor Lee (nine years old) and Nathan Lee (eight years old).

Just as acute inflammation is key for healing and for survival, chronic inflammation is a gateway to chronic disease. Such is the double-edged sword we all must carry: you need inflammation in order to heal and live, but too much for too long can be fatal—or at the very least, accelerate your aging process.

Chronic inflammation will launch you onto the "slippery slope" of a process known as oxidative stress, which causes your body to produce free radicals (toxic chemicals) that can damage all components of your cells, including the cell membrane, proteins in the cell and your precious DNA.

Damage to your DNA will accelerate your aging process. And, damage to your DNA's critical tumor suppressor genes allows for tumor formation, which leads to cancer.

So, now that you know chronic inflammation results in...

...accelerated aging, chronic disease and cancer...

...are you motivated to read this book and learn how to reduce chronic inflammation, regain your energy, feel good and look younger?

Second Edition Update

After receiving some wonderful comments about this book from my patients and other doctors, I decided to update it with their encouraging testimonials and insightful suggestions. For example, I have met several doctors at international medical conferences who mentioned the book, and some of them said they wished I had written more on testosterone therapy in women. So, this edition of Feel Good Look Younger *now addresses that topic as well. In addition, I wanted to update the book with the latest data on protecting your DNA through hormonal balance and proper nutrition. Also, as you may have noticed on the previous page, some artwork from my sons Connor and Nathan, who are in elementary school, is now included as well. I am especially proud of this new edition, and hope you find it even more educational and inspirational for improving your health. Enjoy!*

1

Leaky Gut

You are what you absorb.

A common quote regarding health is, "You are what you eat." However, I prefer to say, "You are what you absorb." After all, your gut is where you either absorb or pass the good, and the bad, from everything you eat and drink.

When you think about it, your gut is much more than just a stomach. It is a nonstop pathway, beginning at your mouth, continuing through approximately 22 feet of small bowel and five feet of large bowel, and ending at your anus. On average, the amount of time it takes—from eating something to having a bowel movement—will be about 24 hours in a normal, healthy individual.

Everything that happens along this 24-hour journey through the gut is vital to your body's 100 trillion cells. Each and every one of those cells will be absorbing their nutrition from what you consume.

Unfortunately, due to affordability, addiction or convenience, too many people consume large amounts of fast foods and processed foods. This, in turn, leads to their body's 100 trillion cells absorbing the chemicals, pesticides, toxins and herbicides that come along with all those fast and processed foods. Consequently, many of today's health problems—ranging from tiredness and obesity, to heart disease—exist (occur) because your cells also have the saying, "You are what you absorb."

It's the Journey, Not the Destination

The three stages along your gut's pathway are: digestion, absorption and elimination. It starts with digestion from chewing and swallowing the food, and then the stomach acid breaking down the food in your stomach.

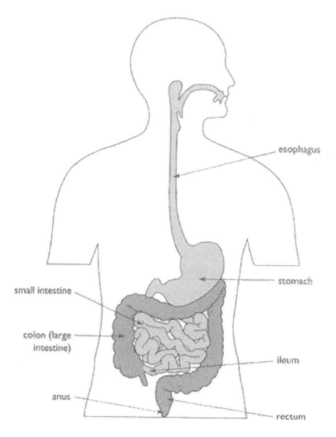

As the food you consume moves through your gastrointestinal tract, digestive juices and enzymes are introduced at specific stages that allow for the absorption of nutrients.

The absorption of nutrients, vitamins, minerals, electrolytes, amino acids and fats takes place primarily in your small intestine. The elimination stage takes place in your large intestine, or colon, and it exits via the anus.

While your intestines' primary job is to absorb and transport the vitamins, minerals and other nutrients from the food you eat through the intestinal lining and into the bloodstream, your intestines also serves as a barrier to prevent the reabsorption of any toxins back into your blood. This is why it is important to have a daily bowel movement and thereby eliminate the toxins out of the body. Otherwise, if elimination is delayed, the toxins will soon be reabsorbed back into the body.

If your gut wall's lining becomes injured or damaged, then a leaky gut can develop. Intestinal hyperpermeability is another name for leaky gut, but I prefer the term leaky gut because it creates a mental image, which makes it easier to understand. Plus, it's just easier to say. Except of course for that one time when I mistakenly replaced "gut" with "butt."

Some doctors dislike the phrase leaky gut because they feel that this condition does not actually exist, or that there is not enough scientific data to support it. However, the current medical literature and scientific data do in fact exist, and will be addressed throughout this chapter.

Leaky gut is defined as an injury to the intestinal wall causing a microscope hole in the intestines that can allow toxins back into the blood stream. Other things that can leak back into the blood system are: bacteria, yeast, fungus, undigested proteins and waste materials. This reabsorption of toxins and other things may be the underlying cause of autoimmune disease.

"I thought my life was over."

When I met Dr. Lee in February 2012, I had been through so many doctors' offices and hospitals, I had lost all hope. I was 20 years old and was recently married when it started happening. Soon, I had lost my job, and my place in college.

During those three years before it all fell apart, drugs and steroids were what held me together. I never knew I would pay for it with the beginning stages of osteopenia, hair loss and gaining almost forty pounds. I started to believe that no one was ever going to help me heal completely. At the last hospital I was in, before seeing Dr. Lee, I remember telling my mom and husband, "No more prednisone or steroids. If I die, then I will let the Lord take me. I am not getting any better, and the drugs are killing me, slowly."

When I left the hospital that day, I went straight to Dr. Lee. By that time, I had lost almost all my hair to the point my scalp was showing, my whole body was leaking fluids—making it hard to keep my body temperature right—and my skin was so inflamed, red, itchy, swollen and tight that it was difficult to sit, stand or walk. All I had done for the last three years of my life was sit at home crying and depressed—hurting emotionally and physically, with no energy. I didn't even want to go outside because of how terrible I felt and looked... at age 20!

My first meeting with Dr. Lee was unlike any other doctor appointment I had ever experienced. It was so totally different, I didn't know what I had got myself into. Yet, I just didn't feel he could do anything for me because, in the past I had just been passed from doctor to doctor, only to again be told they couldn't help me, and that I would just half to deal with it.

After talking with Dr. Lee, he immediately determined I had a leaky gut. Then, after extensive blood work, we knew he was right. The testing showed I had a leaky gut, some hormone issues, and was very sensitive to gluten and quite a few other foods.

So, after several months of changing my diet completely, a lot of IV treatments and detoxing, I started noticing some differences in my body. I started getting my energy back, my hair was starting to come back, and every day, my skin was getting better and better. I was so amazed that all this time it was what I was putting in my body that was harming me—so much to the point, I thought I was going to die.

My whole life, all I ever wanted to do is become a nurse and help people. Now, I have undeniably learned that through nutrition, you really can change yourself for the better. I thank God that my mom found Dr. Lee, and that we gave him a chance. He is the best thing that could ever have happened to me. He has helped me so much. He is a very compassionate person, who truly cares about his patients and their health.

Now, after seeing him for a little over a year, my overall whole body is so much better—inside and out. I remember in the beginning, when I didn't think anything would heal me, that Dr. Lee told me he was going to get me better, and that I'm like a radio who just needs to be tuned the right way. After hearing that, I knew I was in the right place. His staff was also very helpful and resourceful, and very good at making me feel important. Even when I knew how awful I looked, there was no judgment—unlike other doctors' offices I had been to.

I thank God, Dr. Lee, my husband and family, and my friends and church for supporting me all the way. Prayer is a powerful thing, and optimal health—as I am learning from Dr. Lee—is also very important for my body to live a healthy life. Thank you so much Dr. Lee for giving me my life back!

— Lindsey York

A Leaky Gut is the Gateway to Chronic Disease

Again, leaky gut is a condition where there is an injury to the intestinal wall. An intestine is a long hollow tube that allows small molecules (vitamins, electrolytes, water, amino acids, minerals and other nutrients) into your blood system. When there is an injury to the intestinal wall, this allows the larger molecules to leak into your blood system. Normally, the large molecules have no access into your blood system; however, with a leaky gut, such access is granted.

There are several toxic substances that can damage your gut wall. A commonly prescribed over the counter medication to prevent heart disease and stroke is aspirin. However, aspirin has been linked to intestinal hyperpermeability.[1-2]

Non-steroidal anti-inflammatory drugs (NSAID) are a class of drugs that can help with reducing pain and fever and the most popular ones are ibuprofen, naproxen and aspirin. NSAID are the most common medication taken worldwide, and they have been shown to cause leaky gut.[3-4]

Currently, the concept that certain foods can cause leaky gut has not been widely accepted in traditional or conventional medicine. More of this will be discussed in the next section, but certain foods that may be healthy for you may actually cause harm, or even cause a leaky gut.[5-7]

Other causes of leaky gut are the consumption of alcohol, prolonged antibiotic use, chemotherapy, radiation and other toxins.[8-12]

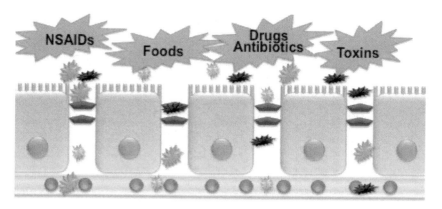

As illustrated (at the cellular level), the causes of leaky gut—NSAIDs (non-steroidal anti-inflammatory drugs), certain foods, drugs, antibiotics and toxins—are absorbed between the intestinal cells and then inadvertently "leaked" out into the blood system. In a healthy gut, only the nutrients are absorbed between the intestinal cells and then passed into the blood system.

Zonulin

In between all intestinal cells are vital little pieces of cellular real estate known simply as "tight junctions." These critical spaces between intestinal cells are responsible for maintaining the barrier between your gut and your blood supply.

Then, in the late 1990s, at the University of Maryland, Dr. Alessio Fasano discovered zonulin, and soon identified it as the "gatekeeper" of your gut—for its unique ability to open up those tight junctions.

Fasano explained that your intestine, with its billions of cells, is your body's largest "gateway." Zonulin is what opens up those billions of gateway spaces between those billions of cells, acting like a gatekeeper and allowing some substances to pass through, while keeping out harmful bacteria and toxins.

Zonulin is produced in your gut, and if it is elevated, then the tight junctions of your gut will open up even more—allowing harmful bacteria and toxins to pass through. Those opened junctions will not close until your zonulin level goes back down. For testing purposes, zonulin can be measured in your blood.[13]

While zonulin is triggered by the certain foods to which you have a sensitivity, there are other triggers for zonulin—and some of these have dire consequences. For example, stress has been shown to increase your production of zonulin, as have: heavy metals, environmental pollutants and toxins, cosmetics, artificial sweeteners, household cleaners, pesticides and other chemicals.

A study with celiac disease patients has also shown that gluten increases zonulin, while another unrelated study has proven that a protein similar to gluten (called gliadin) increases zonulin and leads to a leaky gut as well.[14]

It is important to realize that 70 percent of your immune system is found in your gut, and is known as gut-associated lymphoid tissue (GALT). The gut not only is important for the absorption of your nutrients, but it is also involved with your immune system. The number of white blood cells in the GALT is roughly equivalent to your spleen—an organ that is involved with our immune system. This is why your gut is the largest immune organ in your body.

Also, because your gut is exposed to the external environment (through what you eat and drink), much of it is populated with pathogenic microorganisms. To fight these pathogens, Peyer's patches are located throughout your small intestine. Peyer's patches are critical in the immune surveillance of your intestines, and in facilitating the generation of your body's immune response.

Therefore, when a leaky gut allows "large molecules" (bacteria or undigested food) into your blood system, your immune system will become involved—since it resides in your gut. Because of this, leaky gut has been associated with autoimmune disease.[15-16]

Other Diseases Linked to Leaky Gut

If zonulin is destroyed or damaged, other medical problems—in addition to autoimmune disease—may occur. They include: more inflammation, diabetes, celiac disease, multiple sclerosis, Crohn's disease and cancer.

Diabetes

In 2008, a feature article in Diabetes, *The "Perfect Storm" for Type 1 Diabetes*, discussed the role a leaky gut has in altering the immune system and causing the development of type 1 diabetes. (Type 1 diabetes is an autoimmune disease whereby the body produces antibodies and destroys the production of insulin.)

Remember, the largest organ in your immune system is your gut. The *"Perfect Storm"* article said, "Altered mucosal (gut) immune system has been associated with the disease and is likely a major contributor to the failure to form tolerance, resulting in the autoimmunity that underlies type 1 diabetes."

In another interesting study done on rats that are prone to develop type 1 diabetes, the rats experienced an increase of zonulin levels, which confirmed that leaky gut occurred two to three weeks prior to developing type 1 diabetes. In addition, the rats were given a zonulin inhibitor to reduce the zonulin levels and the results showed that the zonulin inhibitor reduced the incidence of developing diabetes.[17-18]

A 2012 medical study showed that as a marker for leaky gut, zonulin is associated with insulin resistance. Insulin resistance is a medical condition that is a precursor to developing type 2 diabetes. (Type 2 diabetes is the most common type of diabetes, which is when the blood sugar is elevated due to the body not producing enough insulin, or the cells ignoring the insulin. Insulin is necessary for the body to be able to use glucose for energy.)

Another way to think of insulin resistance is that your body is making too much insulin, which will result in becoming fat and developing other serious medical problems. To learn more about the dangers of insulin resistance, please read my book, *Your Best Investment: Secrets to a Healthy Body and Mind.*

As for that 2012 medical study, it proved that higher zonulin levels in the blood are associated with worse insulin resistance. In other words, leaky gut is a precursor of insulin resistance.[19]

Celiac Disease

An autoimmune condition known as celiac disease is when someone's immune system damages the small intestine. Celiac disease can present itself with diarrhea, fatigue, anemia, weight loss or weight gain. Although most people think that celiac disease is caused by gluten, (protein found in wheat, barely and rye) technically it is caused by gliadin (a class of proteins present in wheat and several other grains).

The small hairs, or villi, of the small intestine that are involved with absorption of nutrients are affected, and they actually shrink in size and lose their ability to absorb nutrients. The digestion of gluten/gliadin, leading to the release of zonulin, the onset of the immune system attacking the small bowel and then causing the shrinkage of the small hairs (or villi) of the small intestines, is the mechanism of celiac disease.

The higher zonulin levels (leaky gut) correlated to the severity of celiac disease via a small bowel biopsy. The good news is that once gluten is removed from the diet, serum zonulin levels decrease and the intestine resumes its baseline barrier function. The intestinal damage can heal if gluten is completely removed from the diet.[20-22]

Multiple Sclerosis

An inflammatory and autoimmune disease that attacks the myelin sheaths of the wiring in the brain and the spinal cord, multiple sclerosis is a disease that is more common in women. It can affect the ability to walk, talk, breathe, swallow or even think clearly.

Despite having previously seen the best neurologist in town, one of my patients had a remarkable improvement in her multiple sclerosis when I advised her to eliminate gluten and dairy, and to take bioidentical progesterone since her testing had shown she had a positive food sensitivity to gluten and dairy, and a saliva test had shown she was progesterone deficient. And, because I practice functional medicine (finding the root problem rather than treating a symptom), I recommended that she receive intravenous (IV) nutrition.

The first time she came to see me, she was in a wheel chair. After her fifth IV treatment, she began walking again.

In 1996 there was a paper suggesting that multiple sclerosis was linked to leaky gut. In 2004, at the American Academy of Neurology, a study was presented that there was a correlation of zonulin levels and the severity of multiple sclerosis. Unfortunately, more studies need to be done in this area. I think the gut/brain connection is overlooked in conventional medicine, and that this area needs to be researched heavily—with the goal of one day preventing neurodegenerative diseases.[23-24]

"I really had begun slowing down."

I am 58 years old. I was diagnosed with multiple sclerosis in 2003. By 2007, I really had begun slowing down. By 2009, there were days I could barely move, especially during the summer heat.

In 2010, we found Dr. Lee. He determined that I was lacking in many nutrients and hormone levels. I started with IV therapy. After each IV, I started to feel much better, and I no longer had pain in my legs and feet. After my fifth IV, I started to walk much better. (When I first saw Dr. Lee, I mostly got around in a wheelchair.)

Not only has Dr. Lee helped me feel much better, he has given me a better quality of life. He is truly a caring person.

— *Debra Furino*

Crohn's Disease

An autoimmune disease that is classified as an inflammatory bowel disease, Crohn's disease can affect anything from the mouth to the anus, but usually affects the ileum, which is the final section of the small intestine. Crohn's disease affects about 500,000 Americans, and it can present itself with bloody stool, diarrhea, fever, abdominal pain and weight loss.

I remember a patient who came to see me for a second opinion on his Crohn's disease. He had recently experienced a flareup on his Crohn's disease with blood in his stool, and was hospitalized. He drove three hours one way to see me. He said that he did not want to have surgery, even though surgery had been recommended for his therapy.

After talking to him and doing a workup, he was tested positive for a leaky gut, and had food sensitivities to many foods. With IV nutrition and a program to heal his leaky gut, I was able to get him off most of his medication for Crohn's disease. And, best of all, he no longer needed an operation for his Crohn's disease.

A positive leaky gut test is very useful in patients with Crohn's disease without any symptoms—since this test will precede a clinical flareup of Crohn's disease by as much as one year!

A leaky gut test can also be used in children of parents with Crohn's disease—to screen for developing Crohn's disease. Having a positive leaky gut test, with genetic factors, most likely will be indicative of developing Crohn's disease.[25-28]

"My only prescription was for a healthy lifestyle!"

I was diagnosed with Crohn's disease in 2005. My doctor gave me a steroid and I felt better, without changing any of my habits.

In 2011, I had another strong flareup. I was hospitalized for four days, and I was told I could need surgery. I lost 15 pounds during that time, and it frightened me! My doctors had given me two options: have surgery to remove a part of my small intestine, or go on a drug called HUMIRA®. If I started to take HUMIRA®, I was told I would have to take it for the rest of my life. (I am only 30 years old.) It also had many negative side effects, and was only introduced six years ago. How could I agree to take something for the rest of my life, when it has only been available for the past six years?

Being scared and not sure what to do, I met with Dr. Lee. I am grateful he agreed to meet me right away, because he was my last and only option. After a three-hour evaluation, which no doctor had ever done, he was sure neither surgery nor HUMIRA® was necessary for me. They were both a "bandaid" as he stated. We needed to get to the root cause of why I was having inflammation in my stomach. Dr. Lee gave me the confidence I needed to hear. We did an ALCAT test, and found what foods I was intolerable to. This helped me find out what were some of my triggers. Dr. Lee never prescribed a prescription drug for me—only supplements and vitamins. At first this was new and strange to me—the food I eat, and the supplements I take, are going to be my medicine?

I then returned to receive IV treatments, which helped me recover even faster. If it wasn't for Dr. Lee educating me on how important what I eat is, I know I would not be where I am today. My only prescription was for a healthy lifestyle! I am forever grateful to Dr. Lee. He has changed my life!

— Anthony Hajjar

Cancer

Leaky gut has been associated with many other conditions, but I want to conclude this section with cancer. Unfortunately, I have seen cancer in my previous practice, and have lost some close friends and relatives to cancer.

A recent study noted that a leaky gut may be the root of some cancers. It appears that the hormone receptor known as guanylyl cyclase C (a tumor suppressor), plays a key role in strengthening the body's intestinal barrier. Without this vital receptor, the intestinal barrier weakens, and cancer may form outside the intestine—including the liver lung and lymph nodes.

Dr. Scott Waldman, chairman of the Department of Pharmacology and Experimental Therapeutics at Thomas Jefferson University in Philadelphia is a leading researcher on the guanylyl cyclase C receptor. Dr. Waldman says, "If the intestinal barrier breaks down, it becomes a portal for stuff in the outside world to leak into the inside world. When these worlds collide, it can cause many diseases, like inflammation and cancer."[29]

There are many cancers that, by the time they are diagnosed, it is basically too late for any effective therapy. One example is when someone gets diagnosed with lung cancer. By that time, there is about 15 percent chance of survival in five years.

However, haptoglobin, or a variant of haptoglobin, is a possible early marker for lung cancer. Haptoglobin is an acute phase protein that is released with infection, extreme stress, burns, cancer or injury. Haptoglobin is secreted mostly from the liver, and is also secreted from the lungs, skin and kidneys. Haptoglobin regulates the immune response, binds to free hemoglobin, and prevents the loss of iron and subsequent kidney damage following intravascular hemolysis. Zonulin is a pre-haptoglobin (or comes from haptoglobin 2). In other words, zonulin is the same as haptoglobin. In fact, the terms zonulin and haptoglobin are used interchangeably.[30]

The zonulin pathway is not only found in the gut, but elsewhere in the body—such as the blood brain barrier. In addition to lung cancer, other cancers also have elevated haptoglobin/zonulin levels. They include: bladder cancer, breast cancer, ovarian cancer, lymphoma, leukemia, esophageal squamous cell carcinoma and glioma. These markers look promising in screening for cancers, thereby leading to earlier, more effective, cancer treatments.[31-35]

Diagnosing a Leaky Gut

There are several ways to diagnosis leaky gut, but the classic method is the lactulose/mannitol intestinal permeability challenge test. This test has been used by many medical centers to see if someone has altered gut permeability. Mannitol and lactulose are sugars that are not metabolized by the human body, so they should be excreted by the urine within six hours. Lactulose is one percent absorbed, whereas mannitol is 14 percent absorbed. To diagnose leaky gut, a solution of five grams of lactulose and five grams of mannitol is swallowed, then the urine is collected over six hours. A normal lactulose/mannitol ratio should be 0.03 or less. If it is higher, then the subject has leaky gut.[36]

A relatively new way to diagnosis leaky gut is to determine if zonulin is present, or elevated, in the blood. Remember, zonulin is a relatively new protein discovery that has been shown to control intestinal permeability (the "tight junctions"). Any toxin that injures the intestinal cells can cause a release of zonulin into the blood. If someone has leaky gut, their zonulin will be elevated.[37]

Leaky gut can also be diagnosed by checking for antibodies against zonulin (occludin and actomyosin), which are proteins involved in regulating intestinal permeability. Positive results for occludin and actomyosin are suggestive of a leaky gut.

Another way to diagnosis leaky gut is to have a small bowel biopsy; however, a leaky gut can occur without visible sings on endoscopy. (An endoscopy is a procedure where a scope goes through the nose and down into your small intestines).

However, despite the tissue looking normal on endoscopy, the gold standard test for the small bowel biopsy is to have the sample examined under an electron microscope. An electron microscope is usually located at selective research centers, and this very expensive microscope can reveal the tiny abnormalities that are involved in a leaky gut. Unfortunately, an electron microscope is not available to most doctors or health care providers.

*"People are amazed at my age — asking me to share
my beauty secrets. I just tell them to call Dr. Lee."*

I am a 41-year-old woman who came to Dr. Lee because I was FRUS-TRATED with the following components that were beginning to age me inter-nally, and beginning to show externally: I was tired, had chronic yeast infec-tions, had a short fuse, felt my hormones were out of balance, had bad acne, and my kids were complaining of my smelly bowel movements.

I began to feel much better after my hormones started to become balanced, and when I received IV nutrition (B12 and vitamin D). During my liver cleanse, I noticed that my bowel movements no longer had such a bad odor. After a liver cleanse (I eliminated alcohol, gluten, animal protein, dairy and any processed foods for ten days), when I was reintroducing red meat into my diet, I noticed that I started to feel bad again.

Dr. Lee told me that I have trouble digesting red meat, and one of his initial tests had shown that I have a leaky gut. The amazing thing about Dr. Lee's observation was that before we received the results from the allergy tests he had performed on me, he had already diagnosed me with the same allergies to the same food groups discovered by the allergy tests!

Dr. Lee is outstanding, personable, caring and genuinely easy to speak with. At times I forget he is a doctor! During my first appointment, when I came into his office, he offered me some green tea. I was amazed by this behavior, and even felt suspicious because nowadays, how many doctors sit with you on a comfortable sofa during a consultation and actually listen to you — while understanding what you're saying!

He recognized my body was crying for help. Instinctively, I knew this was a doctor I wanted to treat me. I have recommended Dr. Lee to people I know in need of help. He changes lives. His staff is knowledgeable, attentive, and I TRUST them. After all, Dr. Lee saved my life. I am forever indebted.

Since my gut and hormones have been fixed, it's amazing how good I feel — with extra energy, and my friends are noticing that my skin is looking great. I simply feel balanced now. My gray hair is not as prominent, people are amazed at my age — asking me to share my beauty secrets. I just tell them to call Dr. Lee.

— Nadine Bismark

Food Intolerances

Knowing that the basis for a leaky gut are gaps in the intestinal wall, and knowing that a leaky gut is the gateway for chronic disease, one of the major causes of a leaky gut are food intolerances. However, please understand that although you may have food intolerances, it does not always mean you will have a leaky gut. I have seen patients with many food intolerances, yet they do not develop a leaky gut.

Just as eating healthy helps you feel good and look younger, there could be certain foods you're eating that make you feel tired and look older before your time—actually accelerating your aging process. Not only that, but sometimes, even the healthiest or most organic of food can cause inflammation if you have a food intolerance to that food—which is very different from any food allergy.

This topic is still somewhat controversial since a delayed food allergy can impact any organ in your body with a delayed effect. It can also make this concept hard to follow. In addition, this topic is not yet covered in medical school.

Delayed food sensitivities are, in fact, very different from acute food allergies, which are immunoglobulin E (IgE) mediated. IgE is a certain class of antibody that is involved in the immune system, and an IgE mediated reaction is when the mast cells release chemicals such as histamine, leukotrienes and prostaglandins, which will then cause vasodilatation, or low blood pressure, and also the swelling of the airway. Immediate treatment is required since this is a true medical emergency. Epinephrine is the primary treatment to open the closed airways and to improve the low blood pressure.

Insect bites and eating peanuts are common causes for an IgE mediated acute allergic reaction. The most common acute food allergy that people recognize is a seafood allergy. If someone eats, for example, shrimp, and they have a history of an acute food allergy (IgE mediated) to shrimp, that person is going to suffer from an anaphylactic reaction with the sudden onset and rapid progression of shortness of breath, swelling of the tongue, hives, low blood pressure and swelling that can close the airway.

Delayed food sensitivity, or food intolerance, is a delayed food reaction to a food that is different from IgE. It involves a different part of the immune system separate from IgE. Delayed food reactions will be more chronic and less obvious, with many different symptoms such as: nasal congestion, sinusitis, nausea, headaches, diarrhea, depression, tiredness, heartburn, wheezing and constipation.

Plus, as if to make food intolerances even harder to diagnose, the symptoms do not show up right away. In fact, because food intolerances are not IgE mediated, the symptoms may not show up for several days. Furthermore, if you eat your "allergic" food(s) everyday, or several times a day, the symptoms (like tiredness) may appear chronic.

This is why few people can recognize, in themselves, which foods may be causing their delayed symptoms.[38-39] Delayed food sensitivity has also been associated with asthma, irritable bowel syndrome, chronic hepatitis C infection and inflammatory bowel disease.[40-42]

In fact, when I began to experience some fatigue that was not improving—even after taking a few weeks off from my exercise routine, I suspected food sensitivity. So, just as I usually do with my patients, I started with a saliva test, which showed adrenal fatigue with low cortisol levels.

Based on that, my next test was a delayed food sensitivity test, which revealed that I was highly allergic to mussels and oysters. I had no idea that one of my long-time favorite foods had recently begun causing my fatigue! So I eliminated them from my diet —even though my friends never stopped asking if I wanted to share a dozen oysters as an appetizer—and within two weeks my energy started to ramp back up and I was able to run, cycle and swim again.

In a similar situation, a triathlete patient of mine was complaining of tiredness—even after balancing her hormones, working on her neurotransmitters and optimizing her nutritional support. As it turned out, her delayed food sensitivity was positive for one of her favorite foods—salmon. At that time, she'd been eating it at least four times a week, thinking it was the healthy thing to do.

After eliminating salmon from her diet, her energy returned and she was once again competing—and now winning—in triathlons. Plus, she was able to really enjoy her overall life again. Then, happily, about six months later, she was even able to reintroduce salmon back into her diet once a week without problem.

I use a blood test to see what food sensitivities someone may have. It checks for the cellular delayed hypersensitivity pathway, which is different from the IgG or IgE pathway. There are many companies that offer the delayed food sensitivities with IgG testing. I used to use IgG testing, but you can't really tell if it is elevated if someone has a true reaction versus a recent exposure to a particular food.

Also, I would not get a correlation between the test and the clinical response. For example, one of my teenage patients had the IgG test for delayed sensitivity. Until the results came back, the only advice I could give him for his constant runny nose was to eliminate dairy. After stopping dairy, his nose was dry and he felt significantly better. Later his IgG test came back negative.

Treatment of a Leaky Gut

The 4R Program is what I have successfully used in my practice to treat leaky gut. Developed by Dr. Jeffrey Bland, Chief Science Officer of Metagenics™ and President of Metaproteomics, the 4R Program is designed to promote wellness while healing a leaky gut. The name of the program stands for the four steps in the treatment, which are: Remove, Replace, Reinoculate and Repair.

Remove

Begin by removing the offending agent that is causing the leaky gut. Some common foods or drugs that have been linked to leaky gut are alcohol, ibuprofen, aspirin and caffeine. Or, you may elect to do a food sensitivity test to see if there are certain foods causing a leaky gut.

A food sensitivity test is quicker and more reliable than the process of elimination, which requires someone to determine if they have a reaction (like headache or rash) 24 to 72 hours after eating something. Remember, not everyone with a food sensitivity will have a leaky gut.

Replace

Replace the digestive enzymes, or even the stomach acid, to help digest the food better.

Reinoculate

Reinoculate with beneficial bacteria to reestablish a healthy balance of microflora in the gut. Probiotics are essential, and you can almost never go wrong by taking probiotics. A recent double-blind, randomized study of 150 patients undergoing colorectal surgery had half the group receiving probiotics six days prior to surgery and up to ten days after surgery, while the other group did not receive any probiotics. The probiotic group had lower zonulin levels due to the probiotics (desired effect) and a lower rate of postoperative infection when compared to the placebo group. Other medical studies have also shown the benefits of using probiotics in healing a leaky gut.[43-45]

Repair

Repair the gut wall or lining and support the immune functioning of the gut. Glutamine is an amino acid that has been shown to help repair the gut wall. Glutamine has been studied over 15 years—in studies ranging from the treatment of injuries, trauma, burns, wound healing and sports performance. Glutamine supports and strengthens the gut wall, and protects the GALT tissue.

In addition, nutritional supplements can help assist in decreasing inflammation and help with healing the gut wall. These supplements include: zinc, ginger, rosemary, reduced hops and turmeric. I often use a medical food product that includes all of the above, and it has done wonders for my patients.[46-47]

CHAPTER 1 REVIEW

— The absorption of nutrients, vitamins, minerals, amino acids, fats and electrolytes takes place primarily in the small intestine.

— The intestines serve as a barrier for preventing the reabsorption of toxins back into the blood.

— Leaky gut is an injury to the intestinal wall causing a microscope hole in the intestines that can allow toxins back into the blood stream.

— Causes of leaky gut include: ibuprofen, aspirin, alcohol, drugs, antibiotics, toxins and food sensitivities.

— Leaky gut is associated with: autoimmune disease, more inflammation, diabetes, celiac disease, multiple sclerosis, Crohn's disease and cancer.

— Treat a leaky gut with the 4R Program: Remove, Replace, Reinoculate and Repair.

2

Adrenal Fatigue

Time to bring back the sugar, salt and sex!

One of the analogies I like to use with my patients is that the adrenal glands produce your sugar, salt and sex. The sugar is the cortisol hormone, the salt is the aldosterone hormone and the sex is the DHEA hormone. The adrenals also make catecholamine, more commonly known as adrenaline.

Located above the kidneys, there is a left and a right adrenal gland, and together they look like a triangle-shaped hat. The hormones they produce are vital; yet, until the adrenals begin making too many, or too few, hormones, there is nothing the conventional medical system will do because adrenal fatigue is not yet recognized as a medical condition by mainstream institutions.

And because of that, doctors are trained only in the extreme diseases of the adrenals. One end of the spectrum is where the adrenals make way too much cortisol, which is called Cushing's syndrome. The other end of the spectrum is where the adrenals completely fail and that's known as Addison's disease. Most doctors are not familiar with, nor are they trained in, adrenal fatigue—even though it is the beginning stage of adrenal failure. Part of the reason why most doctors are not familiar with adrenal fatigue is because it does not yet have a specific ICD code for your insurance company to process—which is, unfortunately, why this disease is often looked upon as a condition that does not exist.

I consider adrenal fatigue similar to subclinical hypothyroidism (mild thyroid failure). That condition, unlike mild adrenal failure, is well recognized and widely accepted as a true medical condition. Another similar condition that's accepted is pre-diabetes, glucose intolerance or early diabetes. I truly believe if you're starting to have the early symptoms of a condition, like pre-diabetes, it is much easier to address the condition at that time, rather than later in the chronic stage, which can lead to many complications.

With that in mind, I often tell my patients that treating adrenal fatigue can only make things better—like, "refueling your car." Consider the adrenal glands as the "fuel tank" of your body—which, for the analogy, is like a "car." And when your car is performing poorly, or out of fuel, it's hard to be productive.

Understanding Adrenal Fatigue

Although conventional medicine has yet to accept adrenal fatigue, that doesn't mean it does not exist. Sometimes, as it is with adrenal fatigue, the proof is already out there in medical data, and all you need do is connect the dots. Nonetheless, despite the increasing amount of medical proof, a large medical study to confirm adrenal fatigue has yet to be budgeted by the National Institute of Health (NIH). So, if the NIH is not willing to budget for it, and if the pharmaceutical companies are not going to fund the research—simply because they would have no return on their investment—then this area will continue to be debated.

Shown on the next page is the progression chart of adrenal fatigue. Stage 1 is the hyperstimulation of the adrenal glands to secrete cortisol to handle acute stress. This stage can manifest itself with trouble sleeping, tremors, anxiety and nervousness. Stage 1 is noted to be the alarm reaction or the "flight or fight" response. Stage 2 is when the cortisol levels start dropping and the adrenal glands are unable to keep up with the body's demand for cortisol. Stage 2 is known as the resistance response, and usually presents itself with more insomnia, fatigue and symptoms of an underactive thyroid. Stage 3, where the cortisol output is declining, is called exhaustion. This is a catabolic stage and results in multiple organ system dysfunctions, like the ovarian-adrenal-thyroid axis imbalance. This stage is trying to keep the body surviving while conserving energy. Instead of building up muscle, it starts breaking down muscle or protein for energy—but toxic metabolites are also building up. Stage 4 is where the adrenals are completely exhausted and is known as Addisonian crisis, or acute adrenal insufficiency. Stage 4 is simply known as failure.

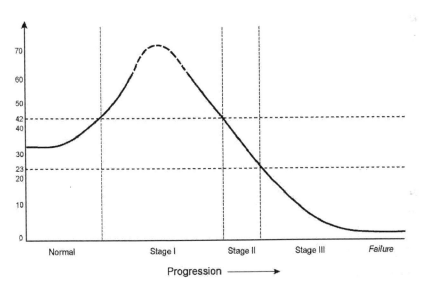

Progression Chart: Stages of Adrenal Fatigue

The length of time in each stage is highly variable. The maximum reported cortisol sum is in excess of 2,000 nM. It is important to note that in all stages of adrenal exhaustion (stages 1, 2 and 3), continued hyperstimulation of the adrenal glands is the common denominator. It is this ongoing hyperstimulation that keeps the body in a state of chronic stress response ("pregnenolone steal" or "cortisol escape"). This is always indicated by an elevated cortisol to DHEA ratio.

Chart © BioHealth® Diagnostics.

The adrenals are regulated by two hormones: CRH (corticotropin releasing hormone) and ACTH (adrenocorticotropic hormone). CRH is produced in the hypothalamus area of the brain and ACTH is produced in the pituitary gland, which is just below the hypothalamus. CRH stimulates ACTH, which in turn stimulates the adrenals to make cortisol. This pathway is known as the HPA or hypothalamic pituitary adrenal axis and was also studied by Dr. Hans Selye when he was investigating the response to stress.

In general, hormones are circulated, or carried, by carrier proteins such as sex hormone-binding globulin (SHBG), cortisol-binding globulin (CBG) and albumin. That is, until they reach the filtration system of the saliva glands. There, while the hormones pass easily through the filtration system of the saliva glands, their carrier proteins are too large to pass on into saliva through this filtration system. This is because the molecular weights of testosterone (288), cortisol, (362), melatonin (232), DHEA (288), estradiol (272) and progesterone (314) are all generally under 400, while the molecular weights of their carrier proteins are very large—albumin is 69,323, CBG is 58,000 and SHBG is approximately more than 100,000. Thus, only the free or unbounded hormones make it into the saliva. No longer attached to their carrier proteins, these particular hormones end their journey in your saliva— where they may now be detected with a saliva test.

In my practice, when I evaluate for adrenal fatigue, I have patients obtain four saliva cortisol levels—before breakfast, before lunch, before dinner and at bedtime. I have seen many different patterns, but the most common pattern I see is that of very low levels for all four cortisol levels. As I mentioned earlier, this is when I tell these patients that cortisol is like fuel, and you're running on an empty gas tank.

To better understand this concept, let's look at several interesting recent medical studies on the hypothalamus pituitary adrenal (HPA) axis and the correlation of low cortisol levels with tiredness.

A 2010 study was done on 33 patients, giving them alpha interferon plus Ribavirin (for patients with hepatitis). Half the group received the medicine and the other group did not receive the medicine. The group that received the alpha interferon with Ribavirin experienced hypothalamus pituitary adrenal (HPA) axis changes with lower cortisol levels (significant flattening of ACTH), which is associated with more fatigue and depression.[1-2]

In another study on patients with chronic fatigue syndrome, it was noted that there was an HPA axis dysfunction with low cortisol levels. This study looked at eight years of published data and determined that low cortisol level and HPA axis dysfunction contribute to fatigue.[3]

Again, more research is needed in this area to confirm this aspect of adrenal fatigue; however, there is current and relative data showing that HPA axis dysfunction and low cortisol levels do in fact contribute to fatigue.

"By the time I went to my appointment, I felt as if my entire body was failing"

Before I met Dr. Lee, I was living a life no one should ever live. I worked from home as a financial trader, which was a good thing and a bad thing. The good thing was that I worked for myself. The bad thing was that I worked by myself. It made my life unbearable as I never left my home, I was alone the majority of the time, and when I wasn't trading, I was asleep, depressed and had no energy. I would cry and not understand why, and I wouldn't even leave my house for food—I was asking my friends to drop off food at my house—when just a year earlier I was very active and loved to go to the gym and even did pilates.

I went to my family doctor and gynecologist, but they could not figure out why I felt so bad. All they wanted to do was put me on anti-depressants, but I would not take them. When a friend referred me to Dr. Lee, I really didn't want to see another doctor. But my friend, who is a doctor himself, kept telling me how good he felt because of Dr. Lee's care, so I decided to give him a try.

By the time I went to my appointment, I felt as if my entire body was failing. Dr. Lee did some advanced testing and learned that I was suffering from severe adrenal fatigue. He also found that I had a very low progesterone level, and one of the lowest vitamin D levels he had ever seen!

Now, all I can say is WOW! He changed my life! I'm on bioidentical hormones and I've reversed my tiredness and I'm enjoying life again. I can't remember when I've ever felt this good. Dr. Lee also figured out my vitamin deficiencies and other imbalances. Then he got me to eat healthier and I lost some weight.

Plus, thanks to my improved health and natural supplements, I no longer take any medication for high blood pressure. Dr. Lee truly changed my life— he is amazing!

— Gina Lowe

Causes of Adrenal Fatigue

I truly believe that you have to take care of yourself by eating healthy, exercising daily, sleeping well, getting your hormones balanced and doing liver detox on a regular basis. Family, faith, friends and being flexible are also important for leading a balanced life. Everything after that is relative.

However, when adrenal fatigue does occur, it is usually because of stress, lack of sleep, environmental toxins, insulin resistance, chronic infections or overtraining (sport or exercise related).

Stress

Most of us consider stress as having too many responsibilities and too little time to complete them. In 1936, Dr. Hans Selye—an endocrinologist, by the way—originated the physiologic view of stress. His discovery of the stress response in rats (via harmful stimuli) showed that the adrenal glands increased in size and thereby increased levels of cortisol, while the thymus regressed, causing a change in the immune system and ulcers, which are very common in today's stressful society.

I see so many of my patients who have been exhausted by a job that pushes them to their limits, family problems, finances and other reasons. The lust of wanting more in life (material things, promotions, fame or whatever it is) does not help.

After a close doctor friend of mine recently died from a stroke at the age of 47, my eyes opened up to what was truly important in life. He was one of the smartest people I ever knew. He spoke four languages and had the gift to remember things in great detail—such as reciting full passages from books he had read decades earlier. My only regret was that I wished we had spent more time together. Life is a precious gift that, all too often, is taken from us by stress.

Lack of Sleep

Apart from having too much stress in life, the lack of good sleep is a cause of adrenal fatigue that I frequently see in my practice. And, like I always say to my patients, "No matter how much I do to treat your adrenal fatigue, you will never fully recover from adrenal fatigue if you don't sleep well."

Many of my patients do not sleep well—whether it is from being unable to fall asleep, or being able to stay asleep. Some unfortunate people even have both problems. I have a set of patients who struggle with sleep. They are wired and tired, and cannot turn off their brains due to the stress in their lives. However, with some natural supplements and hormonal therapy, they regain their sleep quality and feel much better.

Your body needs to heal while you sleep. Also, that is when your growth hormone development is at its highest. That is why good sleep is so important—so our adrenals, brain and the rest of the body can be recharged, renewed and ready for a new day.

Environmental Toxins

Another growing cause of adrenal fatigue is environmental toxins. In conventional medicine, it is acceptable to diagnose and treat toxicity to Tylenol®, ethanol, carbon monoxide, methanol, poisoning or overdose. However, when it comes to heavy metal toxicity, this topic is not readily accepted in the medical community.

Heavy metal toxicity can be a source of chronic inflammation; however, the only heavy metal toxicity that is currently accepted in conventional medicine is lead toxicity, which can affect the heart, bones, intestines, kidneys, reproductive and nervous systems. Lead toxicity can cause permanent learning and behavior disorders in children, and it can cause irritability, headaches, seizures and death.

While there are many heavy metals that can cause tiredness or chronic disease, the most common are: lead (old paint, leaded gasoline, etc.), mercury (certain fish, amalgam dental fillings, etc), cadmium (industrial waste, insecticides, etc.) and aluminum (certain cookware, over the counter antacids, etc.).

Heavy metals may enter through skin contact, breathing or by eating foods or drinking water contaminated with heavy metals. Since heavy metals are stored in body fat, unprovoked urine or blood tests will not detect the presence of lead unless the exposure is recent. Therefore, the most accurate way to diagnosis heavy metal toxicity is by provoking it with DMSA (dimercaptosuccinic acid) or other agents—thereby releasing the heavy metals from the body fat.

Insulin Resistance

A diet that is heavy or excessive in carbohydrates and sugar can produce too much insulin. Too much insulin will cause obesity or belly fat. The overproduction of insulin will cause the body to be stressed, and will lead to a serious medical condition called insulin resistance. To learn more about insulin resistance, please read my book entitled, *Your Best Investment: Secrets to a Healthy Body and Mind*.

Chronic Infections

Other causes of adrenal fatigue include chronic infections, such as Lyme disease, viral infections and parasite infections. For example, I had a patient with adrenal fatigue and chronic sinus infections. He had seen several ear, nose and throat specialists, and their traditional therapies had all failed. By the time he saw me, he had dark circles under his eyes and was totally exhausted. His delayed food sensitivity testing came back positive for everything he ate every day for breakfast —eggs, dairy and yeast. His saliva test showed that he had adrenal fatigue. After cleaning up his diet and using EPA:DHA (omega-3), along with a natural antihistamine, he was able to sleep eight hours without waking up in the middle of the night. He has done very well, simply by reducing his chronic inflammation and getting eight hours of undisturbed sleep every night.

Regarding parasite infections, the parasites come in all sizes, shapes and stages of development—and they can all be a source of chronic infection, which will only contribute to chronic inflammation and thus, adrenal fatigue.

One of the most common domestic sources of parasitic infection is from someones' own pets. Other ways include: eating contaminated food, walking barefoot outside or drinking contaminated water.

So, even though it is true that most parasitic infections occur while visiting developing countries, some of my patients with parasitic infections have never traveled outside the United States. For example, one of them was raised on a farm and grew up drinking well water, while another grew up running barefoot outside constantly.

One common parasite is the pinworm, which can cause anal itching —usually at night since that is when the female lays her eggs near the anus. Other parasites are the roundworm, hookworm and tapeworm, just to name a few. Although a parasitic infection usually presents itself with chronic diarrhea, it can present with chronic constipation.

Stool testing is the best way to diagnose a parasitic infection; however, if you live in a warm climate and the stool has to be mailed or even sent across town, the heat may destroy the parasite infection, causing the test to come back negative for a parasite infection.

Although I see many patients in my office for adrenal fatigue, I usually do not offer stool testing on the initial visit. However, if a patient on the first visit strongly requests a stool test, then I usually grant their wish. The test I prefer to use is from a company that uses DNA probes for the 15 most common parasitic infections, so it does not matter if the parasite is dead or alive upon arrival at the lab.

Overtraining

Before becoming a father, I used to compete heavily in triathlons—including an Ironman distance triathlon. With years of training, combined with a background in swimming and cycling, I was hooked on this sport. (Now, with my young boys, I'm happy just to keep in shape and do one sprint, or one Olympic distance race, a year.)

Thanks to my triathlon background, I'm better able to understand the effects of overtraining in my endurance athlete patients—professionals and top amateurs with adrenal fatigue due to overtraining, which has been proven to burn out the adrenal glands.[4] As a physician, I cure their adrenal fatigue. As a former triathlete, I provide personal insight on avoiding any reoccurrence of adrenal burnout from overtraining.

Leaky Gut

There are many other causes of adrenal fatigue, but the last topic I want to mention here is leaky gut. Leaky gut is an injury to the intestinal wall resulting in a microscope hole, or holes, in the intestines that can allow toxins back into the blood stream. For more information on leaky gut, please see Chapter 1.

"I was almost in adrenal failure."

I am 56 years old, I have been a pharmaceutical sales representative for 31 years and I have been a patient of Dr. Lee's for about 7 years. Initially, I started seeing him for a thyroid condition due to surgery. I will never forget my first visit with him because I quickly found out that he was a very different physician in many ways. Dr. Lee is very compassionate, and he has the desire to listen to what I have to say about what is bothering me.

I've struggled with my weight and being tired all of the time due to my thyroid, or so I thought. Little did I know there was much more that could be contributing to the source of my complaints. Dr. Lee is very meticulous with his decisions, and he did some very innovative tests on me that have literally changed my life. He then worked to meticulously adjust and readjust my medications to keep my levels where they should be. He has also done an energy balance test on my metabolism, a complete hormone test and a complete work-up on my body's levels of vitamins, minerals and amino acids.

In each case, the tests proved insightful results, and the hormone test literally saved my life because I was almost in adrenal failure. After the results of each test, Dr. Lee was able to make the necessary changes for my body's needs—which are different from anyone else's. Dr. Lee did my first-ever hormone test on me to measure my hormones in January 2008. Just imagine, I am 56 years old and no one had ever measured my hormone levels! I have come to find out just how powerful the hormones in our bodies are and how they are responsible for more than I ever imagined. I complained of being tired all the time, and my hormones played a huge role in those symptoms.

Dr. Lee is on the cutting edge of medicine in finding the problems, providing the solutions and not just prescribing medicine to mask the symptoms. He always has the, "Let's find the problem, and then we will try to fix the problem," kind of attitude. I think he loves the challenge. When I found out he was leaving Gessler Clinic to open the Institute for Hormonal Balance, I was in a panic because I knew he had made such a huge difference in my life, the quality of my life and my well-being that I didn't want to lose any of the progress we'd made by trying to find another physician. I had decided I was going to follow him as patient wherever he went, even if I had to put a mortgage on my house to do the traveling! I was relieved to find out he would only be one hour away. I am very fortunate to have a physician like Dr. Lee, and I know there will be many success stories of other people he will help by making a difference in their quality of life, just like he has done for me.

— Jacqueline Smith

Treatment of Adrenal Fatigue

The treatment for adrenal fatigue is typically straightforward—once you know the cause; however, finding the cause may at times prove difficult.

The first step is to achieve quality sleep. I often use natural supplements like melatonin, theanine (Amino acid) GABA (a brain chemical that has a relaxing effect), chamomile, magnesium, valerian, and others. I sometimes use bioidentical progesterone in men to help with their anxiety. Usually, most of my patients do very well when they start to sleep better, and are getting undisturbed sleep.

Another part of treating adrenal fatigue is the reduction of mental or emotional stress. Sometimes, this is the hardest part because, "It's not so much what you're eating, but what's eating you." I say that to my patients because, while I can diagnose what foods they should or shouldn't be eating, I can't always help with what's "eating" at them. Factors such as family, financial or work stress may play a significant role in this regard, as well as everyday stress. Any of these stressors may very well trigger the adrenals to secrete high levels of cortisol.

For example, a study in patients undergoing same day surgery has shown an elevated cortisol level.[5] Additionally, a recent study has shown an association of high cortisol levels with depression.[6] To counteract this, the use of phosphatidylserine has been shown to lower high cortisol levels.[7-8]

Taking progesterone at night has helped many of my patients relax and sleep better. (See Chapter 5 for more information on progesterone.) Occasionally, I have resorted to short-term use of Ativan® or Valium. Another way to relax is with Ashwagandha, a wonderful adaptogenic herb that helps lower high cortisol levels. Ashwagandha is a herb often used in ayurveda medicine, an Indian system of holistic medicine, to help cope with physical and emotional stress. Ashwagandha is also known as winter cherry or Indian ginseng.

Other aspects of the treatment of adrenal fatigue include: cleaning up the diet (focusing more on fiber, less on sugar), the avoidance of foods that cause any delayed food sensitivities (which will lower chronic inflammation), lowering high blood sugars through lifestyle modification, and taking extra nutrients either by mouth or intravenously.

As for supplements, in my practice I may use rhodiola rosea, B-complex vitamins, vitamin C, or pregnenolone with or without DHEA or adrenal extract. Occasionally, I've had to use bioidentical cortisol for the short-term to restore any extremely low cortisol levels.

However, the overall most effective way for the adrenals to improve is through intravenous (IV) nutrition. (See Chapter 10 on IV nutrition for more information.)

"Upon having my adrenal gland removed, I started to feel extremely depressed."

I want to say that Dr. Lee has really helped tremendously. I first saw Dr. Lee four months after having one of my adrenal glands removed. Upon having my adrenal gland removed, I started to feel extremely depressed. Before the surgery, I used to enjoy going to church, but after the surgery I felt too tired and just lost interest. In addition, I was suffering from terrible hot flashes. I started to cry a lot and started to gain weight. I felt that I was losing control of my life.

After seeing Dr. Lee, he mentioned that my hormones were not balanced after my one adrenal gland was removed. After starting natural hormonal therapy I stopped crying, my energy significantly improved and I am attending church again. I'm enjoying life once again and I feel like I'm back to my old self. Also, my hot flashes disappeared. Dr. Lee, you are the greatest.

— Martha J. Timms

CHAPTER 2 REVIEW

— Adrenal fatigue is a common cause for tiredness. It is a condition where the adrenal glands are failing and unable to make adequate hormones—primarily, cortisol.

— Adrenal fatigue, unfortunately, is not yet accepted in conventional medicine; therefore, it does not have a specific code for insurance companies to process.

— The best test to check for adrenal fatigue is a 4-panel (morning, lunch, dinner and bedtime) saliva test.

— The underlying causes for adrenal fatigue are numerous; yet, all of the causes are linked to chronic inflammation. Some examples of those causes are: diet that is high in refined sugars, leaky gut, chronic infection, parasite infection, food sensitivity, obesity, heavy metal toxicity, mental stress or excessive exercise (such as ultra marathoners and long distance triathletes).

— The basic treatment for adrenal fatigue includes: reduce chronic inflammation (or, treat the underlying cause), reduce stress, sleep for eight undisturbed hours every night, reduce insulin levels by eating more fiber and vegetables, increase lifestyle activity and take supplements that restore the adrenal glands.

3

HYPOTHYROIDISM

**Be sure you're fueled up
before stepping on your accelerator.**

Reasonable estimates currently show that ten percent of the U.S. population has hypothyroidism (underactive thyroid disease). This means there are nearly 30 million Americans with an underactive thyroid—more than the number of Americans with diabetes (24 million) or cancer (11 million)!

Situated in the front of your neck—just below the muscle layers—your thyroid gland, which is shaped like a butterfly with its two wings being the left and right thyroid lobes, which wrap around your trachea. The sole function of your thyroid gland is to take iodine, found in many foods, and convert it into the thyroid hormones: thyroxine (T4) and triiodothyronine (T3).

Thyroid cells are the only cells in your body able to absorb iodine, which they use to combine with the amino acid tyrosine to make T3 and T4, which are then released into the bloodstream and are transported throughout your body where they control metabolism (the conversion of oxygen and calories into energy). Every cell in your body—let me repeat that—every cell in your body, depends on your thyroid hormones for the regulation of your metabolism.

To best illustrate this important point, I'll build upon the "your-body-as-a-car" analogy from the previous chapter. I like to use this analogy as a way of explaining to my patients how adrenal fatigue (low cortisol) is like driving a car with very little fuel in the tank. You can keep on driving with your "fuel light on" (your body's warning signs, like chronic tiredness); but, pretty soon your fuel will be gone (adrenal glands exhausted) and no matter how much you step on that accelerator (push your thyroid), you're not going anywhere until the tow truck shows up and brings you to the "mechanic" (me), and I refill your tank with its precious fuel.

Underactive Thyroid

Hypothyroidism (underactive thyroid) upsets the normal balance of chemical reactions in your body, creating a condition in which your thyroid gland doesn't produce enough of certain important hormones. Women, especially those older than 50, are more likely to have hypothyroidism. It seldom causes symptoms in the early stages, but over time, untreated hypothyroidism can cause a number of health problems, such as obesity, joint pain, infertility and heart disease.

"Other doctors simply prescribed thyroid medicine and sent me on my way."

Before becoming a patient of Dr Lee's, other doctors simply prescribed thyroid medicine and sent me on my way. For years (I'm 53 now), no one listened to my complaints of, "this isn't right yet... I'm still so tired... I'm feeling drained."

Dr Lee's depth of knowledge, of both the medicines and the physiological workings of the body, has given me back good health, enabling me to live my life with energy—with a "full tank of gas." Tracking all the components of thyroid functions, including T3, and looking at the whole picture of what I personally need to stay healthy, is what I most appreciate about Dr Lee.

— Marie Magrath

Now, at this point, I need to explain thyroid-stimulating hormone (TSH). Your thyroid is regulated by TSH, and TSH is measured in your blood with a standard test that monitors your thyroid. TSH is produced in the pituitary gland (in the brain). Now, for the confusing part: TSH is regulated by another hormone called thyrotropin releasing hormone (TRH). Although TSH and TRH look the same, they are two different hormones. TRH is produced in the hypothalamus gland (also in the brain, and positioned above the pituitary gland).

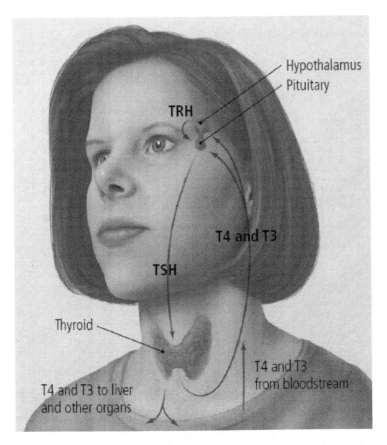

Under ideal conditions, the hypothalamus will send a signal in the form of thyrotropin-releasing hormone (TRH) that enables the pituitary gland to secrete thyroid-stimulating hormone (TSH). In response, the thyroid gland releases T4 and a small amount of T3 into the blood stream.

Currently, there is a debate among thyroid experts on what is considered a normal level for TSH. While your TSH level is an excellent screening tool (in the form of a blood test) for a thyroid disorder, exactly what is considered normal may vary.

In fact, over the last 30 years, the normal reference range for TSH had been lowered to where most laboratories were using a level of 0.3 to 5 mU/L for normal. Then, in 2005, Dr. Leonard Wartofsky, one of the leading experts in thyroid disease, presented evidence that a TSH less than 2.5 mU/L should be normal.[1] Therefore, a TSH above 2.5 mU/L indicates that you most likely have an underactive thyroid condition, especially if you have symptoms of underactive thyroid.

"I didn't like the cranky, irrational and moody person I was turning into."

I have been under the care of Dr. Lee for a little over a year for treatment of hypothyroidism. When I first began my treatment I was lethargic, depressed and overweight. I was unhappy with the way I felt overall, and I didn't like the cranky, irrational and moody person I was turning into.

Dr. Lee changed the thyroid medication I was taking from a synthetic hormone to porcine thyroid and it has made quite a difference. I lost 15 pounds, am now a regular at the gym, and have the energy to stay awake later in the evening. I feel better about the way I look, feel and, most importantly, the way I interact with the people who matter most to me in the world... my family.

— Kirsten Kostur

Symptoms of an underactive thyroid include tiredness, weakness, dry skin, slow speech, cold insensitivity, memory impairment, constipation, depression, weight gain, loss of hair, swelling and decreased sweating. Additionally, if you have a family history of underactive thyroid, you're at risk of developing hypothyroidism.

The most common underactive thyroid condition is Hashimoto's thyroiditis—an autoimmune thyroid condition in which your immune system starts destroying your thyroid. A positive thyroid antibody test like a thyroglobulin antibody or thyroid peroxidase antibody level with an elevated TSH indicates the presence of Hashimoto's thyroiditis.

Thyroxine (T4) and Triiodothyronine (T3)

Your thyroid produces and secretes thyroid hormone that is about 90 percent T4 and 10 percent T3; however, T3 possesses about four times the hormone "strength" as T4. Most of your T4 and T3 are bound to proteins like albumin and thyroxine binding globulin. Only a small percentage is not bound, and therefore called Free T4 or Free T3. These free hormones are the only ones that are hormonally active. Most of your T3 is produced from the conversion of T4 to T3 in the liver. In this regard, T4 can be looked upon as a pro-hormone for T3.

T4 has four iodine molecules, whereas T3 has three iodine molecules. By removing one iodine molecule in a process called deiodination, T4 can be converted into T3; however, this conversion requires an enzyme called deiodinase. Factors that inhibit the conversion of T4 into T3 are elevated cytokines [bad blood markers: interleukin-1 (IL-1), tumor necrosis factor (TNF) and interleukin-6 (IL-6)], liver disease, renal disease, systemic illness, high cortisol, zinc deficiency, high glucose, selenium deficiency, amiodarone, beta-blockers and steroids.[2]

T4 Versus T3/T4

In the field of endocrinology there is an ongoing debate about the value of using T3 therapy versus the therapy combination of T4 and T3. The standard and current treatment for hypothyroidism has been the use of levothyroxine or T4. A study published in the New England Journal of Medicine has shown that T4 and T3 therapy was beneficial in improving mood and neurophysiological tests.[3] However, there are other studies with different ratios of T4 and T3 that have not shown the benefit of T3 and T4 over T4 therapy alone.[4]

There is much data suggesting that T3 is very valuable in reversing tiredness, improving a weak heart, improving on depression, improving on memory performance, lowering cholesterol and reducing inflammation. Even in the negative study of T4 and T3 therapy versus T4 alone, patients preferred the T4 with T3 combination, to T4 alone.[5] Another negative study showed that T4 and T3 are not any better than T4 alone; however, it was shown that patients preferred T4 with T3.[6] Furthermore, in a review of nine studies comparing T4 versus T3/T4 combination therapy, it was shown that most patients actually prefer the combination therapy.[7]

Over the years, I've followed and reviewed these studies and I've noticed that the studies used low doses of T3, and also that suboptimal levels of Free T3 were achieved. I believe the T4 with T3 debate will continue until these two inconsistencies have been resolved in a well-designed clinical study.

What's In It For You?

The benefits of T3 therapy or low T3 in the medical literature are worth noting. It has even been shown that T3 therapy has improved cardiac contractility, and has helped patients with congestive heart failure.[8] Furthermore, a low Free T3 predicts atrial fibrillation after open heart surgery.[9]

Low T3 is also a strong predictor of health in cardiac patients, and might be directly implicated in poor prognoses for cardiac patients.[10] Then, in a more recent 2008 study, intravenous T3 treatments showed no side effects with arrhythmia, and have helped patients with heart failure by improving cardiac function and lowering their heart rate.[11]

"I began to think my life as I knew it was over."

I am a professional in the community, involved in a career that requires high levels of energy. When I developed Graves' disease and had my thyroid radiated, I began to think my life as I knew it was over. I was constantly lethargic and had no stamina. Synthroid® simply did not work for me.

When I found Dr. Lee, he turned my life around and I am finally my old self again. He worked with me to find the right T3/T4 combination for me. Soon, I lost 35 pounds and my energy soared back to my usual high level.

— Cookie

In fact, a higher risk for heart disease has been associated with mild underactive thyroid disease, and a mild underactive thyroid has even been shown to increase the risk for arrhythmia after open-heart surgery.[12] A recent 2007 study in Norway found that there is a direct relationship with higher blood pressure and a higher TSH. (Remember, a higher TSH means underactive thyroid.) This study was on over 30,000 individuals with high blood pressure (greater than 140/90) with normal TSH. They compared the group with a TSH of 3 to 3.5 mU/liter to the group with a TSH of 0.5 to 0.99 mU/liter and noticed the group with a higher TSH had higher systolic and diastolic blood pressure readings.[13]

Mild underactive thyroid disease is also associated with insulin resistance, which is associated with heart disease.[14] Additionally, in a recent review of the literature with the use of high doses of thyroid medication, there was no bone loss in men or premenopausal women, although it remains unclear with postmenopausal women.[15]

On the other end of the spectrum, the side effects of over-treating underactive thyroid disease are bone loss, irritability, weight loss, heat intolerance, arrhythmia, diarrhea, elevations of liver function tests, hair loss, menstrual irregularities and rarely seizures. The most common concerns are bone loss and arrhythmia.

Most of the medical studies have not shown any bone loss with thyroid replacement. And a study that uses high doses of thyroid medication for the treatment of thyroid cancer showed no bone loss.[16] In a recent review of the literature with the use of high doses of thyroid medication, there was no bone loss in men or premenopausal women, although it remains unclear with postmenopausal women.[17]

In my experience with combining T4 and T3 versus T4 alone, I find that most patients prefer the combination treatment as to T4 alone. Beside the use of T4 and T3, zinc and selenium should also be used to help with an underactive thyroid.

Extra iodine can also help if a patient is iodine deficient. In addition to optimizing the thyroid function (improving the conversion of T4 to T3) one has to reduce chronic inflammation or lower the cytokines (IL-6 and TNF-alpha) and improve on the metabolic syndrome or lower high glucose and high insulin levels. Although the data for combining T4 and T3 over the use of T4 alone has been recently not supportive of any difference, most patients actually preferred the combination of T4 and T3 instead of T4 alone.

"My health improved almost immediately."

I was diagnosed with a thyroid condition and was quite ill. After seeing three doctors, I was finally referred to Dr. Lee, who knew how to treat my illness. My health improved almost immediately and today I am fine. My eyesight has improved to the point where I no longer need to wear glasses for close work, only distance, and my health is great.

— *Nellie Lloyd*

Also, the use of T3 in the clinical studies were very low in dosage and that the goal of achieving a higher Free T3 was not optimized. For some labs, normal Free T3 is 140 to 420 pg/dL. The goal for my patients is to have their Free T3 in the upper range of normal (i.e., 380 to 420 pg/dL) or the top quartile of the Free T3 range without developing any side effects, like tremors or heart palpitations. Monitoring for bone loss with a urinary N-telopeptide test should be done at least twice a year.

Tyrosine

Thyroxine (T4)

Triiodothyronine
(T3)

"Reverse T3"
(inactive)

Thyroid hormones are derivatives of the amino acid tyrosine, which is bound covalently to iodine. The three principal thyroid hormones are thyroxine (T4), triiodothyronine (T3) and Reverse T3. These three hormones differ by the amount of iodine attached to the amino acid tyrosine. T4 has 4 iodine molecules, while T3 and Reverse T3 have 3 iodine molecules.

In hormone therapy, T4 is known as Synthroid®, Levoxyl® or levothyroxine; whereas, T3 is known as cytomel. The combination therapy of T4 and T3 that I use in practice is Armour® Thyroid (a natural desiccated thyroid hormone derived from pig thyroids). The T4 and T3 in Armour® Thyroid is bioidentical to human T4 and T3. Two other combinations of T4 and T3 are Nature-Throid™ or WesThroid™. Nature-Throid™, WesThroid™ and Armour® Thyroid consist of approximately 80 percent T4 and 20 percent T3. Another way to use a combination therapy is to mix levothyroxine (T4) with cytomel (T3). Or, T3 may be used alone. I prefer to use a combination therapy of T4 and T3, and have used multiple combinations of T4 with T3 (for example: 50 percent T4 with 50 percent T3), as well as T3 by itself.

What They Don't (But Should) Teach in Medical School

Reverse T3 is an important hormone that most endocrinologists have not been trained in. I remember that in my endocrinology training at the University of Pittsburgh, we were taught to focus on the TSH, total

T4 and Free T4. Reverse T3 was used only in research and was not available for clinical practice. The thyroid produces about 90 percent T4 and 10 percent T3. T4 is a prehormone (an inactive thyroid hormone that is later converted in peripheral tissues into an active hormone). T4 is converted to either T3 or Reverse T3. Most of this conversion takes place in the liver; although, a small percentage of the conversion can happen in the kidneys, pituitary and thyroid.[18]

The conversion of T4 to T3 is an important step because T3 is the active thyroid hormone. According to an important review article by Dr. Antonio Bianco of the Thyroid Division, Department of Medicine, Brigham and Women's Hospital and Harvard Medical School, until T4 is converted to T3, T4 has no physiological effect because it does not enter the target nucleus at high enough concentrations to bind to the required thyroid receptors. The conversion of T4 to T3 requires a removal of one iodine molecule so that it goes from 4 iodine molecules (T4) to 3 iodine molecules (T3). This step is called the 5' deiodinase or (D1, D2). Reverse T3 is generated by the enzyme 5 deiodinase (D3) converting T4 to Reverse T3.[19]

"I doubt any doctor in Sweden would know how to correct this."

My name is Helen Alfredsson and I am 47-year-old professional golfer from Sweden. I first saw Dr. Lee in 2009 due to my low energy. I initially ranked my energy to be 2/10 and it was progressively getting worse. I have been an athlete my entire life, and I am well-attuned to any changes in my body.

I was noticing that I was also having trouble recovering after my workouts, and that I was having trouble concentrating. Dr. Lee determined that I had a low thyroid with a very high Reverse T3. We have adjusted my thyroid medication several times, and each time my Free T3 improves and my Reverse T3 drops. I doubt any doctor in Sweden would know how to correct this condition—or even how to test for Reverse or Free T3. Since Dr. Lee has been managing my thyroid, my energy, my focus and my recovery from workouts have all been much better. I have been recommending Dr. Lee to all my friends.

— Helen Alfredsson

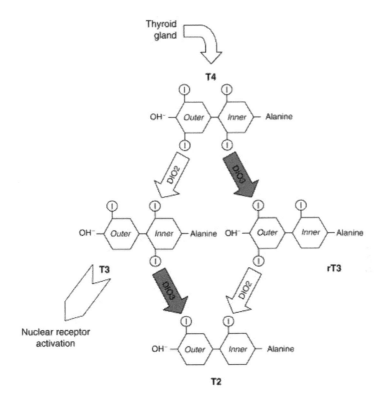

The pathway of T4 (converting to either T3 or Reverse T3) is the principal circulating form of thyroid hormone, but has relatively low biological potency for activation of nuclear TH receptors; however, the potency is increased considerably by the conversion to T3 through outer ring deiodination. This is mediated by type II deiodinase (DIO2). Conversely, T4 can be converted to an inactive form (Reverse T3) by inner ring deiodination mediated by type III deiodinase (DIO3). Both T3 and Reverse T3 can be further metabolised by DIO3 or DIO2, respectively, leading to diiodothyronine (T2) formation.

Because the most common conversion of T4 to T3 happens in the liver, should the liver not function well, then the conversion of T3 is compromised. A study in 1979 showed that patients with chronic liver disease have an elevated Reverse T3 with reduced Free T3. Currently there has been confirmation that some people can have a genetic defect in the D2 or 5'-deiodinase that converts T4 to T3. In a recent study with 552 patients it was found that 16 percent of the study group had an enzyme defect (D2 Thr92Ala), and that this group of people did much better on T4/T3 combination therapy versus T4 therapy.[20-21]

The reason why many of my patients actually feel much better on the combination therapy of T4/T3, or with T3 therapy versus T4 therapy, is due to the genetic defect of converting T4 to the active T3.

When a 5' deiodinase enzyme defect is present—as illustrated—the pathway of T4 will be unable to convert to T3, resulting in a low T3 and a higher Reverse T3.

Another study at the National Institute of Health demonstrated proof that T3 therapy is beneficial. In the study, they took patients with an enzyme defect (D2 Thr92Ala) and gave them TRH (thyrotropin releasing hormone) to see what the thyroid response would be. The results showed a blunted rise in T3 levels. In addition, a 2013 study revealed that when T4 therapy was given to hypothyroidism patients who had the D2 Thr92Ala enzyme defect, the patients developed more central obesity and higher blood pressure.[22-23]

The previous T4/T3 combination study (which did not confirm that T4/T3 combination therapy was better than T4 alone) did not look at genetic polymorphisms (defects) on the (D2) 5' deiodinase enzyme, resulting in problems with converting T4 to T3. The study showed that 16 percent of the patients had this enzyme (D2) defect. There is also the issue of the low dose of T3 therapy that was used in the previous studies. More studies need to be done to look at either T4/T3 or T3 alone—especially in patients with the D2 Thr92Ala enzyme defect (which means they cannot covert T4 to T3) to confirm beyond doubt that T4 therapy is not the gold standard for the treatment of underactive thyroid.[24]

I also look at the Reverse T3 and the Free T3/Reverse T3 ratio. Although there is not yet much medical data, I find this insight very important. An elevated Reverse T3 is not helpful since this is an inactive thyroid hormone. The goal is to have a higher Free T3 over a Reverse T3. I see many patients who have seen other thyroid specialists and are not feeling well—despite a normal TSH. With those patients, I try to optimize the Free T3 and lower the Reverse T3. There are some natural supplements to help lower Reverse T3.

Summary

In summary, to reverse tiredness you have to optimize the thyroid condition with the use of T4 and T3, or T3 by itself, while monitoring for any potential side effects. If the TSH is suppressed to less than 0.3 mU/ml, then you need to be monitored twice a year for bone loss with a urinary N-telopeptide test. In addition, reducing chronic inflammation and replacing any zinc, selenium or iodine deficiency will significantly help optimize the underactive thyroid.

I usually avoid the use of iodine replacement with patients with positive thyroid peroxidase antibody—since this will accelerate thyroid failure. However, before addressing the thyroid, you need to always address any adrenal fatigue first. Or, as in the car analogy, be sure you're fueled up (fix your adrenal fatigue) before stepping on your accelerator (your thyroid).

"There is a big difference between "normal" and "optimal" hormone levels."

Prior to seeing Dr. Lee, I was struggling with steady weight gain, low body temperature, thinning hair, chronic insomnia, fatigue and debilitating PMS. I am 34 years old, and had seen several doctors about these issues (before Dr. Lee), none of them recognized that I had a thyroid problem. Although my TSH was only mildly elevated, Dr. Lee's more thorough testing revealed that I was definitely hypothyroid with low Free T3 and very high Reverse T3.

To correct my problem, he prescribed cytomel (T3 hormone). Due to some other endocrine issues, it took me a while to work my way up to the right dose of cytomel, but my patience paid off! Now I feel much better than I have in years! Unlike many doctors I've seen over the years, Dr. Lee keeps up with new research and is willing to think and act beyond conventional medical dogma. He also has a great attitude, emphasizes a healthy lifestyle, and approaches his patients as a partner in their health care.

After working with Dr. Lee for almost two years, it has become obvious to me that there is a big difference between "normal" and "optimal" hormone levels, especially when it comes to quality of life. I really appreciate that Dr. Lee always focuses on optimal.

— S. Sparks

CHAPTER 3 REVIEW

— Before optimizing your thyroid gland, you first need to address adrenal fatigue, which is why I often say in my practice, "Be sure you're 'fueled up' (adrenal fatigue has been corrected) before stepping on your 'accelerator' (thyroid)."

— Have your doctor check your thyroid peroxidase antibody and thyroglobulin antibody to see if you have an autoimmune thyroid problem. Also, request a Free T3 test—not to be confused with a T3 Uptake, which is commonly entered incorrectly into the computer by lab technicians or heath care providers.

— Find a physician that is comfortable in the use of T4 and T3 therapy.

— Optimize your Free T3 level to the top quarter of the reference range. You'll need to be monitored by blood test, and also be warned about the side effects of taking too much T3 or T4—which are: fast heart rate, bone loss, stroke, arrhythmia, diarrhea, weight loss, heat intolerance, liver failure, hair loss, menstrual irregularities and seizures (rarely).

— Correcting a sluggish thyroid can help with: tiredness, weakness, dry skin, slow speech, cold intolerance, memory, constipation, depression and weight loss.

— If you have an elevated Reverse T3, then you need to do a liver detox (see Chapter 11), or have your thyroid medication adjusted to lower your T4 and increase your T3.

4

ESTROGEN

**As always, the operative word here is "bioidentical,"
as opposed to "synthetic."**

Does it not surprise you to read that when most people think of hormones, they think of estrogen? Estrogen is a beautiful hormone with many incredible benefits, that I will discuss later; however, estrogen has received some bad press lately, having been linked with breast cancer, stroke and heart disease since the 2002 Women's Health Initiative (WHI) study.

Yet, a very important point of the study was that animal-derived estrogen with *synthetic* progesterone—not *bioidentical* hormones— was associated with breast cancer, stroke and heart disease. There is a huge difference between animal-derived estrogen and bioidentical estrogen, which I will address in detail.

Since the WHI study came out, the mere mention of estrogen has been tainted. After about five years of the WHI trial, researchers stopped the trial early due to a higher incidence of heart disease, stroke, breast cancer and lung clots compared to women on a placebo. Dr. Jacques Rossouw, director of the National Institutes of Health, which headed the WHI study summarized the findings, "The WHI results tell us that during one year, among 10,000 postmenopausal women with a uterus (as opposed to those who have had their uterus removed) who are taking estrogen plus progestin, eight more will have invasive breast cancer, seven more will have a heart attack, eight more will have a stroke and 18 more will have blood clots, including eight with blood clots in the lungs, than will a similar group of 10,000 women not taking these hormones. This is a relatively small annual increase in risk for an individual woman.[1-2]"

The media seized upon the theme that all estrogen therapy is harmful, and did not differentiate (or even acknowledge any differences) between synthetic versus bioidentical estrogen. Because of the WHI study, most doctors—who consider this study as the gold standard for hormone replacement therapy—now believe that all estrogens are harmful. The results of the WHI on the use of animal-derived estrogen (which is derived from pregnant horse urine) and synthetic progesterone showed higher rates of heart disease, stroke and breast cancer. The animal-derived estrogen that was used in the WHI study was conjugated equine estrogen, otherwise known as Premarin® (as in "pregnant mare urine"). The conjugated equine estrogen is produced from pregnant horse urine and is still the standard medical care to use for postmenopausal women, despite the results of the WHI study. Hands down...

...the WHI study has proven that synthetic hormones are not safe.

Although some people consider Premarin® to be "natural," or bioidentical, since it is collected from pregnant horse urine and not produced in a laboratory that alters the chemical structure of the estrogen, it is not bioidentical to humans—horses, yes, people, no. Premarin® has many horse estrogens that people do not have. Also, the enzymes needed to breakdown Premarin® may be lacking in people. Because of these reasons, and because so many women do not feel well with it, I consider Premarin® as a synthetic hormone that is not natural, or bioidentical, to the human body.

Around the same time the WHI study came out, another similar study came out from France showing that hormone replacement therapy with bioidentical estrogen and progesterone is safe, and that it does not increase the risk for breast cancer—as always, the operative word here is "bioidentical," as opposed to "synthetic." Bioidentical hormones are identical in molecular structure to the hormones that we make, whereas synthetic hormones are chemically altered and are therefore not identical in molecular structure to any hormone that we make.

The 3,175 postmenopausal women in the French study used bioidentical estrogen and progesterone for nearly nine years and proved that hormonal therapy was safe, improved the quality of life and also did not show an increase risk in breast cancer.[3] This study (Which never made it into the media like the WHI study!) is further proof that if you need to replace a missing hormone, it is crucial to use bioidentical hormones to achieve optimal health.

After the WHI report came out in 2002, the use of Premarin® and Provera® (synthetic progesterone) dropped. Despite the negative fall-out from the WHI study, in the spring of 2003, the FDA granted approval to the makers of Premarin® and Provera® to market low dose versions of Premarin® (0.45 mg) and Provera® (1.5 mg). Now, what I find even more amazing than that is there is no long-term study on these new "low dose" synthetic hormones. I believe if the National Institutes of Health funds a long term study on these "low dose" hormones, they would get similar negative results. All I can do is ask, "Why would you use a synthetic hormone that has been linked to cancer, heart disease, blood clots and strokes, when you can use bioidentical hormones?"

"And why not, when you just feel good!"

Thank you Dr. Lee for making me feel great! After years of suffering with migraine headaches and trying to live without hormones, Dr. Lee successfully alleviated my migraines, I have no more hot flashes, and my husband says I am in a much better mood. And why not, when you just feel good!

— *Suzi Olson*

Most of my patients over 45 are on bioidentical estrogen to help with their symptoms of memory loss, help rebuild their bone loss, improve on their libido and help with their vaginal dryness and hot flashes. When there is a decrease in estrogen there is a cascade of events that accelerates the aging process. For example, the skin becomes thinner, drier and wrinkled. Estrogen replacement can reduce dry skin, improve on the elasticity of the skin and reduce skin wrinkling.[4-6]

Estrogen is also helpful in lowering blood sugars, improving on HDL (good cholesterol), lowering cholesterol and improving on insulin resistance.[7-8] In addition, bioidentical estrogen can help with memory loss by activating cholinergic neurons in the brain.[9-10] Further studies need to be done to confirm that estrogen can help prevent dementia. Animal-derived estrogen, or the horse estrogen that was used in the WHI study, failed to help protect brain function; in fact, it actually lowered brain function. Estrogen is also important in building strong bones. However the timing of estrogen is important to prevent osteoporosis. The key is to start early and not wait until it's too late.[11]

Bioidentical Estrogen and Heart Disease

The leading cause of death for women who live beyond menopause is heart disease. It is estimated that women over 45 will die of heart disease ten times more often than of breast cancer. Heart disease increases rapidly after menopause, whereas the rate of breast cancer increases slowly.[12] The American Heart Association lists the modifiable risk factors for heart disease as high blood pressure, high cholesterol, smoking, physical inactivity, stress, obesity, alcohol abuse and diabetes.

Unfortunately, the American Heart Association (AHA) does not recommend estrogen replacement.[13] The reason is that the ten studies the AHA reviewed were all on animal-derived estrogen and synthetic progesterone, and showed that these synthetics were not protective for heart disease. The studies were not on bioidentical hormones. So once again, the confusion of hormonal replacement continues.

The good news is that bioidentical estrogen improves cardiovascular risk factors, lowers cholesterol, increases the good cholesterol and improves on lowering blood sugars.[14-15] Further studies need to be done to confirm that early bioidentical estrogen and progesterone replacement reduces heart disease. Yet, with the current data that's out there, early bioidentical estrogen replacement is definitely crucial in the prevention of cardiovascular disease.

"I know how to listen to my body now."

I went through early menopause at 28 years of age. That was over 20 years ago, and I was put on hormone replacement therapy; however, I only took the drugs for about a year. I was always sick to my stomach and had severe headaches, so I chose to stop the drugs on my own. I was confused as to what to do for hormone replacement and felt there was not enough data on what effects these drugs could have on me, so I did not take any drugs for over 20 years.

At 50, I began having symptoms of fatigue, brain fog, weight gain and no energy. I had already gone through the normal symptoms of menopause—night sweats, hot flashes, short temper—years before. But now, I began experiencing hip joint pain, lower back pain, knee joint pain, leg cramps and shin splints.

Then one day, just over a year ago, I had finally had enough. I went to Dr. Lee to see if he could customize a hormonal balance program that would work for me. He conducted numerous tests and determined that I had osteopenia bone density, low calcium, low vitamin D levels and low progesterone levels. He also did an MRI on my brain and found a pituitary tumor—which was probably the cause of my early menopause. He customized a plan for me that treated me with proper nutrition, vitamins and natural hormones. I am so grateful for his guidance and helping me achieve hormonal balance in my life. I now feel that I can live my life to the fullest. I know how to listen to my body now, and I will continue to follow proper nutrition, healthy eating and a proper exercise program. Thank you Dr. Lee for helping me see the light.

— Carolyn Accola

The Nuts and Bolts of Estrogen

Aside from whether estrogen is synthetic or bioidentical, there is also the issue of how it is administered. Currently, most of the published medical studies on estrogen have been on oral estrogen—despite the fact that estrogen given by mouth has been linked to other problems. Taking estrogen orally has been shown to increase inflammation and increase the inflammatory markers of CRP, IL-6 and TNF (bad blood markers). Conversely, taking estrogen through the skin does not increase the inflammatory markers.[16-17]

Since oral estrogen has been shown to increase inflammation, it is also linked to blood clots. Whereas taking estrogen through the skin (via transdermal delivery) has been shown to have less of a risk for blood clots.[18-19] Taking estrogen by mouth lowers a very important hormone, insulin-like growth factor-1 or IGF-1. This is the last thing you want to do if you want to improve on energy. Lowering IGF-1 accelerates the aging process. Taking estrogen through the skin, however, does not lower IGF-1.[20-21] Another effect of oral estrogen is that it raises triglycerides (fat that is different from cholesterol) whereas estrogen given through the skin lowers triglycerides.[22] Taking estrogen by mouth will eventually go into the liver and induce clotting factors, inflammatory markers and other proteins that can increase the risk for heart disease, stroke and accelerate the aging process. Replacing bioidentical estrogen through the skin or under the tongue (sublingual) that bypasses the liver is strongly recommended.

My experience with bioidentical estrogen replacement is that most of my patients have a sense of improved energy and vitality. In a study of postmenopausal women after three months of transdermal estrogen treatment, the women showed improvement in anxiety, positive well-being, vitality, hot flashes, sweating and libido.[23] Estrogen interestingly improves hot flashes by raising the body's thermostat in sweating.[24] In addition to feeling better and having more energy, estrogen is believed to be one of the many reasons women typically live longer than men.[25]

While estrogen is the predominate hormone in women, it is also produced in men—just at lower levels. Estrogen is a large hormone in size and is produced from the ovary, adrenals and also from the fat cells.

Now, not to make it confusing, but you do not produce only one estrogen. For simplicity sake, I often explain this by saying there are three different types of estrogen that you make: estrone (E1) is the estrogen of menopause, estradiol (E2) is the estrogen of youth and estriol (E3) is the estrogen of pregnancy. To better understand the differences between bioidentical estrogen and animal-derived estrogen, you first need to understand the differences between the three estrogens that your body produces.

17β-Estradiol   Estriol

Estrione

Illustration of the differences between the three estrogen: estradiol, estriol and estrone. (17B-estradiol is the same as estradiol.)

Estradiol (E2)

Estradiol levels stay high in the bloodstream during the teenage years until it starts decreasing around the 30s, and then totally disappearing after menopause. Estradiol is the estrogen of youth that helps the brain form memory, helps bones become stronger and helps protect the heart from heart disease.[26]

Estriol (E3)

Estriol levels are extremely elevated during pregnancy. After pregnancy, estriol levels drop and estradiol again takes over. Estriol helps with the baby's development and also plays a protective role against breast cancer during pregnancy.[27] Estriol has been considered in conventional medicine to be a weak estrogen or ineffective estrogen and it has not been widely used in conventional medicine. The estrogen that is still used a lot in conventional medicine is conjugated equine estrogen or the "pregnant mare estrogen."

The use of estriol is the best choice for hormonal replacement since estriol has never been associated with any cancer activity in humans and has even been shown to prevent breast cancer. (Low estriol levels have been shown to be a risk factor for breast cancer.[28])

According to the American Cancer Society, Asian women have the lowest rates of breast cancer in the world. Also, studies have shown that Asian women have the highest estriol levels during pregnancy, which may have a protective role in preventing breast cancer.[29] In a Norwegian study it was even noted in a group of women using an estriol-containing preparation that it was not associated with a higher risk of breast cancer.[30]

Although estriol-like substances are now being patented to treat and prevent breast cancer, and there is data suggesting that estriol is the preferred estrogen, future large studies on estriol and breast cancer are needed.[31-34]

Estrone (E1)

Estrone is the estrogen of menopause. During menopause the production of estradiol from the ovary has stopped, and estrone is made from the conversion of the male hormones (androstenedione) that is produced from the adrenal glands. The conversion to estrone usually occurs in the fat cells but it can occur in the breast, muscle, liver or bone.[35] Estrone is the major source of estrogen in postmenopausal women, and estrone does help with bone formation.[36] However, high levels of estrone are associated with breast cancer.[37] And unfortunately, there are hormones containing estrone that are still being sold, such as estropipate, which is a modified estrone—despite the fact that estrone has been linked to breast cancer.

Estrone can be converted to estradiol by an enzyme called 17 beta-hydroxysteroid dehydrogenase type 1 (17HSD type 1) and estradiol can convert to estrone by an enzyme called 17 beta-hydroxysteroid dehydrogenase type 2 (17HSD type 2).[38]

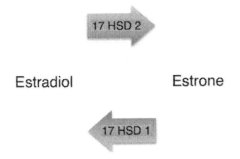

Illustration of the conversion of Estradiol to Estrone by the enzyme 17 beta-hydroxysteroid dehydrogenase type 2 and the conversion of Estrone to Estradiol by the enzyme 17 beta-hydroxysteroid dehydrogenase type 1.

Estrone can also break down into other estrogen metabolites. One noteworthy theory for the cause of breast cancer is that there is an over-expression of the 17 HSD type 1 enzyme—which makes more estradiol in the breast tissue—with the highest rate of breast cancer being diagnosed in postmenopausal women with an average age of 61.[39]

Estrone can then be converted into estradiol in the breast tissue by the 17 HSD type 1 enzyme, which can then feed on the breast cancer cells to become more aggressive. Inhibitors of this enzyme in breast tissues are being looked at for future treatment of breast cancer.[40-42]

Estrogen binds with two different receptors: estrogen receptor alpha (ER-alpha) and estrogen receptor beta (ER-beta). There are estrogen receptors in almost every part of the body: brain, heart, kidney, blood vessels, bone, lung, intestine, prostate, endometrium and breast.[43] ER-alpha promotes breast cell proliferation while ER-beta inhibits proliferation and prevents cancer development.[44] Estradiol equally activates ER-alpha and ER-beta while, in contrast, estriol selectively binds to ER-beta, which is believed to help protect from breast cancer.[45] This combination of estradiol and estriol has the unique ability to protect against breast tissue from overstimulation of the ER-beta receptor.[46] Again, future studies on the combination of estradiol and estriol, or the use of estriol alone, on breast cancer are needed.

Prempro® Proven Unsafe in 2002...
Premarin® Proven Unsafe in 2004

The most common animal-derived estrogen that has been used to treat postmenopausal symptoms is Premarin® (conjugated equine estrogen), which was introduced in 1942, and is made primarily from— as the three consonants of its name indicate—*pre*gnant *ma*re u*rine*.

Premarin® also has 50 percent of estrone and zero percent of estriol, as well as many different estrogens that are very different from humans. It has equilin, equilenin and dehydroestrone sulfate which are not produced in humans.[47] Premarin® also has been shown to reduce the number of the ER-beta receptors[48]—not a desirable effect!

In addition, the metabolite of conjugated equine estrogen also contains a potent carcinogenic estrogen, 4-hydroxy-equilenin, which promotes cancer by inducing DNA damage.[49-50] With the selective binding to ER-alpha and down regulating the ER-beta receptors, and also the metabolite of 4-hydroxy-equilenin, it is no surprise that Prempro® has been linked to breast cancer. Despite the 2002 WHI report showing Prempro® (animal-derived estrogen with synthetic progesterone) as unsafe and, despite the 2004 WHI study showing Premarin® as unsafe, it is estimated that there are still approximately nine million women still taking Premarin®.[51] Education to health care providers and to all women interested in hormonal replacement is vital for any kind of reform on this matter.

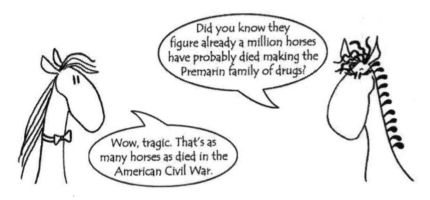

This illustration from an International Fund for Horses campaign draws attention to the cruelty of the Pregnant Mare Urine (PMU) industry, which exists internationally to serve Pfizer. People were encouraged to print and send the campaign flyer to Pfizer to express their distaste for the consequences to women—as well as mares and foals—resulting from a decades-old technology that relies on the increasingly unpopular and detrimental use of pregnant mare's urine (conjugated equine estrogen) to make drugs that have been proven to be cancer-causing for women.
Artwork © Vivian Grant Farrell, March for PMU Horses, International Fund for Horses.

Estrogen given alone in postmenopausal women is associated with a higher risk for endometrial (lining of the uterus) cancer. Thus, estrogen should be given with bioidentical progesterone in postmenopausal women to prevent the risk for endometrial cancer.[52] It is crucial to replace both estrogen and progesterone in women who have had a hysterectomy in order to prevent the condition of estrogen dominance. In regard to the effects of estriol on the endometrium (lining of the uterus), there are studies to show that estriol does not increase the thickening of the endometrium and does not increase the risk of endometrial cancer.[53-55] Many of my postmenopausal women have complaints of vaginal dryness, or vaginitis. Estriol has provided excellent results in resolving these complaints, and estriol has also been used to prevent urinary tract infections.[56]

"To no avail, I tried all the latest gimmicks
to attain my health goals."

I've always been active—maintaining a full-time professional career and enjoying the challenges of the outdoors. But at 55 I began to feel tired, anxious and, quite frankly, on a downhill slide. To no avail, I tried all the latest gimmicks to attain my health goals. Then I read an article regarding Dr. Lee and I decided to try one more time to feel good, have more energy, perform better and continue living healthy.

Within the first three months I was feeling like a new woman! And all Dr. Lee had to do was readjust my bioidentical hormones (Biest and progesterone) and add a supplement—but the most important thing was that he knew exactly what I needed!

Since then, over the past year, I've improved my running time from a 14-minute mile to an 11:14-minute mile. I've participated in all of the Track Shack Races while gleefully comparing my last year results to this year! What a difference! Recently, I completed my first Walt Disney World Half Marathon with energy to spare, and I needed very little recovery time afterwards.

But my greatest achievement occurred on June 23, 2010 when I reached the summit of Half Dome in Yosemite National Park. That particular climb is a total distance of 16 miles out and back, with a total elevation gain of 4,842 feet, a peak elevation of 8,836 feet, and a skill level rating of "extremely strenuous."

I reached the summit in 6 hours, and returned to the comfort of the lodge in
6.5 hours.

   Thank you Dr. Lee—and your team of professionals—for improving my
strength, energy, confidence and most importantly, my life!

                                                        — Marie Schiavi

Estrogen in the Environment

Besides the side effects of animal-derived estrogens, we are
constantly exposed to excess estrogens from our toxic environment.
There is a class of estrogens called xenoestrogens that are not estrogen
in structure, but have estrogen effects. These are fat soluble and non-
biodegradable in nature, and some of the sources are plastic drinking
bottles, sunscreens and lotions. Other sources are birth control pills,
insecticides, weed killers, paints and preservatives that also
contaminate our ecosystem. Also shocking is the effect of
xenoestrogens on our wildlife. Male fish are becoming female fish and
it is believed that the culprit is from industrial and pharmaceutical
chemicals polluting our waterways.[57]

Another major concern is the early sexual development of girls—as
early as eight or nine—due to exposure from environmental estrogens.
The two xenoestrogens at issue are phthalates (plasticizers) and
bisphenol A (commonly known as BPA), which were originally
developed as synthetic hormones, but are now used in all
polycarbonate plastics and the linings of food and beverage cans.[58] All
the more reason as to why it is so crucial to drink water that has been
properly filtered, and to avoid bottled water in BPA containers.

With such constant exposure to exogenous estrogens from our toxic
environment, one is at risk of developing estrogen dominance.
Estrogen dominance is an area of endocrinology that is not yet widely
accepted. The symptoms of estrogen dominance range from anxiety,
irritability, irregular menstrual cycles, heavy menstrual flow, fatigue,
insomnia and mood swings. It usually presents around age 30 to 40
years of age, although I have seen it develop as young as 20.

Estrogen dominance is where there is normal or excessive estrogen with a relatively low progesterone level. The key in treating estrogen dominance is with bioidentical progesterone to balance the ratio of estrogen and progesterone. I commonly see many patients that have had their symptoms treated with antidepressant medications, sedatives or with birth control pills instead of simply being treated with progesterone. In fact, the use of bioidentical progesterone leads to many incredible results, which are covered in the next chapter.

The Breakdown of Estrogen

To screen for breast cancer in women and prostate cancer in men, I offer a 24-hour urine estrogen metabolism test. Estrogen is also produced in men, but in lower levels as compared to women. Estrogen is a fat-soluble hormone (as opposed to a water based hormone) that is metabolized through your liver. Your liver can change the fat based hormone to water based so that it can be eliminated. In other words, your liver is an important place where estrogen is either metabolized or detoxified.

The estrogen can then take the good pathway or the bad pathway—depending on the health of your liver. The breakdown of the estrogen is either sent to the bowel or to the kidneys to be excreted. When stool remains in the bowel for a long time, as in constipation, the estrogen is reabsorbed. The excessive estrogen then increases the stimulation of breast tissue, leading to an increased risk for breast cancer.

It has also been shown that high levels of the 16 alpha hydroxylated estrogens (bad estrogen that is excreted from the liver) increase the risk of breast cancer.[59] In a recent 2009 study, it was shown that high levels of the 16 alpha hydroxylated estrogens increase the risk of breast cancer.[60] Another study showed that lower levels of the 16 alpha hydroxylated estrogen lowers the risk of breast cancer.[61] A simple test to screen for breast and prostate cancer (although it is not the only cause for breast or prostate cancer) is a 24-hour urine test to look at the ratio of the good estrogen and bad estrogen (2-hydroxyestrone/

16alpha-hydroxyestrone ratio). This test also looks at how the liver is metabolizing or detoxifying the estrogen. If one has undesirable levels of the 16-hydroxylated or 16alpha-hydroxyestrone estrogens, then there are natural ways to convert those bad estrogens to the good estrogens.

Besides screening with a 24-hour urine test to look at the ratio of good estrogen and bad estrogen (2-hydroxyestrone/16alpha-hydroxyestrone ratio), you can reduce the chance of breast cancer by increasing the enzyme known as quinone reductase. Quinones are organic compounds that are naturally found in the environment and in our body. However, quinones can rapidly form into free radicals that cause oxidative damage to our cells. Quinone reductase is an important enzyme in neutralizing quinones. One mechanism of breast cancer is the production of estrogen quinones that can cause DNA damage and later transform breast cells into cancer cells.[62]

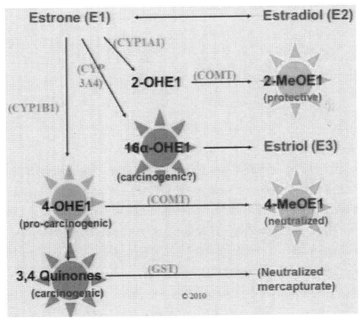

Diagram of the breakdown of estrogen. Estrone can be broken down into many metabolites. The protective metabolites are the 2 MeOE1 (2-methoxyestrone), Estriol and 4 Me-OE1(4-methoxyestrone).

Artwork © Genova Diagnostics®

There is now evidence that women with a defective quinone reductase do poorly with surviving breast cancer.[63] Fortunately, there are natural supplements that can increase your quinone reductase, such as: epigallocatechin gallate (green tea is an excellent source), resveratrol, gamma-tocotrienol (vitamin E is an excellent source), alpha-lipoic acid and glutathione to name a few.[64-67] I recommend that my patients drink green tea and take resveratrol and vitamin E to increase their quinone reductase, and for their excellent antioxidant properties.

As mentioned earlier, estrogen given orally has a risk for heart disease, stroke, clotting and causing blood clots in the lungs and legs.[68] Transdermal estrogen has no negative effect on clotting. Conjugated equine estrogen or "horse estrogen" has been shown to show an increase in clotting.[69] Thus, estrogen should not be given orally since it can increase the risk of clotting, increase triglycerides, and lower IGF-1 (insulin-like growth factor-1). Lowering IGF-1 will accelerate the aging process, and cause one to be fatigued.[70] Therefore, estrogen should always be given by a cream or patch (transdermally), or under the tongue (sublingually), so it will bypass the liver.

Estrogen Benefits

The benefits of estrogen are to prevent memory loss, promote bone health and reduce heart disease. The FDA has approved bioidentical estradiol, such as Climara®, Vivelle-Dot® and Estraderm®, and I occasionally prescribe the bioidentical estrogens listed; however, I prefer to prescribe sublingual or topical (transdermal) applications of the combination of estradiol and estriol—otherwise known as Biest, which can be made by a compound pharmacist.

Biest is 80 percent estriol and 20 percent estradiol. For example a dose of Biest of 1 mg has 0.8 mg of estriol and 0.2 mg of estradiol. I also use estriol under the tongue or vaginally. Estriol needs to be made by a compound pharmacist. It is important to check for the metabolism of estrogen in the urine to screen for breast cancer and to use the lowest dose possible. Also, it is prudent that every woman follow through with her routine mammogram and also breast examination.

Another important piece of advice for preventing breast cancer is to increase your intake of green tea, alpha-lipoic acid, vitamin E and glutathione in order to increase your body's quinone reductase enzyme.

Estrogen, overall, is heavily debated and more long-term studies are needed to answer its many questions. There are differences in the types of estrogen (estrone, estradiol and estriol), synthetic versus bioidentical, the route of administration, different estrogen receptors and the use of bioidentical progesterone versus synthetic progesterone (progestins), that need to be addressed with human clinical trials.

Although I think it may take another ten years for a full change, the tide is definitely beginning to change for the management of menopause in women with a personal or family history of clotting. Thanks to the recent acceptance of bioidentical hormones in a 2012 article referencing the North American Menopause Society, the Endocrine Society, the International Menopause Society and the European Menopause and Andropause Society—which now all contain positive statements regarding both transdermal (patch) estradiol and micronized progesterone (not progestins)—it was concluded that the use of transdermal (patch) estradiol and the use of bioidentical progesterone could possibly reduce breast cancer, stroke, clots and gallstones.[71]

Another recent medical study also demonstrated the benefits of bioidentical hormones on healthy postmenopausal women's breast tissue. This study compared the use of bioidentical hormones versus the synthetic hormones (horse estrogen with synthetic progesterone). The use of bioidentical hormones with estradiol gel (1.5 mg daily for two 28 day cycles) and oral micronized progesterone (200 mg per day for the last 14 days per cycle) did not increase the gene expression of KI-67 gene for breast cancer; whereas, the synthetic hormones significantly increased the KI-67 gene, and also increased the breast density on mammography.[72]

Without a doubt, unopposed estrogen increases the risk of endometrial cancer, so it is highly recommended to use progesterone in the treatment of postmenopausal women. Since there is a small increase in the risk of breast cancer, heart disease and stroke with the use of animal-derived estrogen with synthetic progesterone, it is prudent to use only bioidentical estradiol, bioidentical estriol and bioidentical progesterone in hormonal replacement therapy.

Estrogen Replacement Protecting DNA

The most important structure of your body is your DNA. Every cell in your body, except for red blood cells, has DNA. The ends, or caps, of your DNA are called telomeres, and they are the protective part of your DNA. As you age, the length of your telomeres will shorten. This shortening process will reach a critical point where your telomeres shorten to the tipping point. At this tipping point, if there are excessive free radicals or oxidative damage to the cell—where the telomeres can no longer protect the DNA—then DNA damage will begin, and you will experience premature aging, chronic disease, cancer and early death due to DNA damage. In other words, telomere length has been correlated with the aging process.[73-74]

In a study of 130 postmenopausal women, half the group received hormonal therapy with estrogen and progesterone. The study showed that the women who received hormonal therapy for more than five years had significantly longer telomere lengths when compared to women who did not receive hormonal therapy. This study showed that hormonal therapy slowed down the aging process.[75]

And, in a recent study on mice, it was shown that estrogen deficiency is associated with shorter telomere lengths, and that estrogen replacement increases telomere lengths.[76]

"We've always prided ourselves on
staying healthy, young and very active."

My husband, Batista, and I are both in our early 70s. We've always prided ourselves on staying healthy, young and very active in running the business we started together in 1958—owning a hotel and a five-star dining facility.

Over the last few years, we'd both become increasingly tired. Knowing of Dr. Lee and his Institute for Hormonal Balance through our daughter, we made appointments. Dr. Lee, to my dismay, informed me that I was deficient in several hormones! He immediately started me with IV therapy on a weekly basis and on low doses of bioidentical hormones on a daily basis. Today, I have never felt better since I was in my teens!

Dr. Lee is a miracle worker, extremely intelligent, empathetic and he truly seeks out ways to reverse the natural changes that occur as we age! Batista and I will always be extremely grateful and thankful to Dr. Lee for all of the wonderful things he is doing for us, and for all of his patients!

— Evelyn Madonia

CHAPTER 4 REVIEW

— Estrogen comes in three "flavors," which are estrone, estradiol and estriol. If you need estrogen then you should take bioidentical estrogen that has estradiol and/or estriol. You should not take estrogen alone (without also taking progesterone) or else you may become estrogen dominant.

— Avoid taking estrogen by mouth or by pill since this will increase the clotting factors from your liver and thereby increase your risk for blood clots, strokes and heart disease. In addition, taking estrogen by mouth accelerates your aging process by lowering your insulin-growth factor-1 (IGF-1), which is a very important hormone.

— I recommend that every person over the age of 30 be screened for breast cancer (in women) or prostate cancer (in men) by doing a 24-hour urine estrogen metabolism test. This test looks at your ratio of good estrogen to bad estrogen (2-hydroxyestrone/16alpha-hydroxyestrone ratio), which is how your liver breaks down estrogen. It's a great test to see if you have a "weak liver."

— Avoid using horse-derived estrogen (Premarin®) since it is not a natural human ovarian estrogen.

— Taking bioidentical estrogen can help a woman with vaginal dryness, low libido and hot flashes. Bioidentical estrogen will also lower cholesterol and blood sugars, while improving memory, energy and well-being.

5

PROGESTERONE

Synthetic progestins can stimulate breast cancer, whereas bioidentical progesterone can protect from breast cancer.

As one of the first hormones to become deficient, progesterone is produced by both men and women; however, women produce larger amounts as it is involved with the menstrual cycle, pregnancy and embryogenesis. Progesterone is produced in the ovaries, placenta and adrenal glands. Progesterone, like estrogen and testosterone, is derived from cholesterol.

Before I begin with this section on progesterone deficiency, a quick review of the menstrual cycle is in order. Which reminds me of a time when I was with a mother and her teenage son, and he obviously did not want to hear anything about his mom's cycle, so the mom looked at him and plainly said, "You need to learn this," and she was right. It is true that most teenage boys—and men—have no idea how a female reproductive cycle works.

For a woman in her reproductive years, the menstrual cycle is about one month long. If pregnancy does not occur, then each month she will have a period. Most women will have a period that lasts about five days. There are three stages of the menstrual cycle. The first part is called the follicular phase, and is where the estrogen level starts rising to help the uterus (womb, or where the fetus lives in during development) lining to thicken up. The second part is the ovulation, or the release of the egg from the ovary. Some women know exactly when they ovulate since they can feel it. The third phase is the luteal phase, where the progesterone rises. Progesterone causes the uterus lining to secrete a special protein to help prepare for implanting of the fertilized egg (sperm is needed to fertilize the egg). If there is no implantation of a fertilized egg, then the thickened uterus lining falls apart and a period will follow.

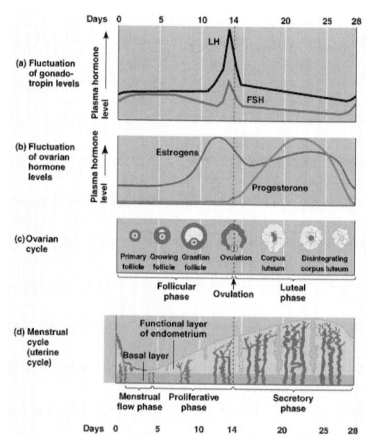

The first part of the female menstrual cycle is the follicular phase (days 1-13), the second part is the ovulation, or release of the egg (days 13-14), and the third part of the cycle is the luteal phase, where the uterus is thickening up in preparation for the implantation of a fertilized egg (days 15-27).

The monthly menstrual cycle is repeated until pregnancy (after which, it resumes), menopause or when the ovaries stop working (due to certain medications that shut down the ovaries, or by surgical removal of the ovaries).

Progesterone deficiency usually begins around the age of 35, although I have seen its onset in teens. Progesterone deficiency starts before estrogen deficiency, and usually presents itself with: irregular periods, insomnia, irritability, weight gain, tiredness, low libido and hot flashes.

Progesterone at its correct levels has the ability to reduce anxiety, as well as improve upon sleep quality, libido, hot flashes, migraine headaches and mood swings. It also can decrease the risk for breast and prostate cancer, improve on protecting the brain and help with lowering cholesterol.

The most common progesterone-related complaints I hear from my female patients are irritability, anger, mood swings, worsening of insomnia and, "I used to be this calm person and now I'm an emotional basket case!"

Although progesterone was discovered about 70 years ago, its therapeutic potential is far from being realized. The only problem with progesterone is the confusion of bioidentical progesterone with synthetic progesterone (known as progestin). And while progestin and progesterone may sound the same, they are very, very different.

By adding an extra chemical to progesterone, the pharmaceutical companies are modifying progesterone, thereby creating synthetic progesterone. The only reason pharmaceutical companies modify the already perfect progesterone into synthetic progesterone is so they can patent it! Never mind that by doing so, they've altered its chemical structure, made it synthetic, and are selling something that has been shown to increase the risk of breast cancer, heart disease and stroke.

Progestins are synthetic progesterone. Progestins increase your risk of dementia, heart disease, stroke, breast cancer and blood clots. Some examples of synthetic progesterone are Provera®, medroxyprogesterone, Mirena® (Intrauterine devise, IUD) and birth control pills. In fact,

Provera®, medroxyprogesterone, has been associated with higher rates of breast cancer, heart disease, stroke and blood clots. I strongly advise against the use of Provera®, medroxyprogesterone.

As shown in the illustration below, the difference between bioidentical progesterone and synthetic progesterone is significant. The top structure (progesterone) is bioidentical, and the bottom structure (medroxyprogesterone) is synthetic progesterone. You can plainly see that they are not the same. It is such a shame that the media, and especially health professionals, still get this concept confused.

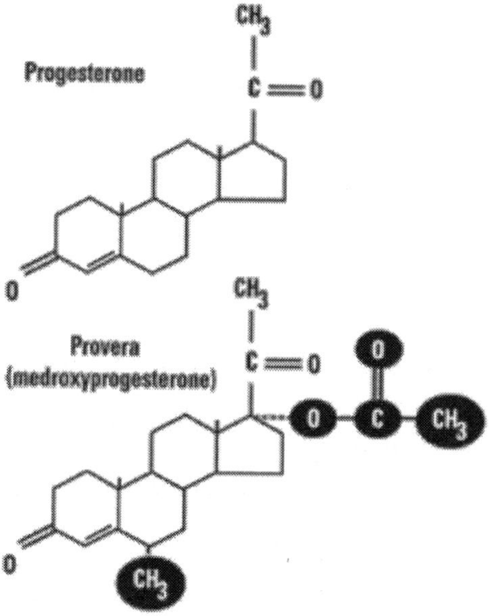

When viewed as a chemical structure, the differences between bioidentical progesterone and synthetic progesterone (medroxyprogesterone) are obvious.

Then, along with the negative effects caused by progestins, the bioidentical progesterone gets undeservedly associated with the synthetic progesterone.[1-2]

An excellent example of the pervasiveness of the confusion on hormonal replacement came about when one of my nurses said that she was progressively not feeling well, couldn't sleep, had anxiety, was depressed and didn't enjoy her Saturday morning golf anymore.

So I checked her hormones and as it turned out, she had estrogen and progesterone deficiency, and was in adrenal fatigue. Soon after treatment with bioidentical hormones she made a 180-degree turn and resolved all her symptoms. Later she saw two other doctors for unrelated issues and was told by both doctors that the hormones she was on can cause breast cancer, heart disease and stroke. She just smiled and said politely, "Yes it can, with synthetic hormones, but I'm on bioidentical hormones."

At this point I'd be remiss if I didn't make reference to a position statement from the Endocrine Society® saying there is little to no evidence to support the claim that bioidentical hormones are safer or more effective than the commonly used synthetic versions of hormone replacement therapy.[3] However, I am respectfully adamant that there actually is a significant amount of data that does in fact substantiate a difference.

Dr. Holtorf's Rebuttal

For example, an excellent rebuttal to the Endocrine Society® position statement is a 2009 paper written by Dr. Kent Holtorf.[4] For his paper, Dr. Holtorf exhaustively evaluated 196 research articles in order to say, "A thorough review of the medical literature supports the claim that bioidentical hormones have some distinctly different, often opposite, physiological effects to those of their synthetic counterparts."

Dr. Holtorf went on to reference study after study on breast cancer, heart disease, heart attack and stroke to show that, "Substantial scientific and medical evidence demonstrates that bioidentical hormones are safer and more efficacious forms of HRT (hormone replacement therapy) than commonly used synthetic versions."

Regarding the effects of progesterone and synthetic progestins on breast tissue, Dr. Holtorf provided evidence that, "Synthetic progestins have potential anti-apoptotic (anti-apoptosis is the property—like in cancer cells—with the ability to live forever) effects and may significantly increase estrogen-stimulated breast cell mitotic activity and proliferation. In contrast, progesterone actually inhibits estrogen-stimulated breast epithelial cells (this is a desired effect, which is achieved with bioidentical progesterone).

Progesterone also downregulates estrogen receptor-1 (ER-1) in the breast, induces breast cancer cell apoptosis, diminishes breast cell mitotic activity and arrests human breast cancer cells." In other words...

...synthetic progestins can stimulate breast cancer, whereas bioidentical progesterone can protect from breast cancer.[5-7]

In addition, for women undergoing hysterectomy, bioidentical progesterone helps prevent fibroids and/or endometriosis.

Furthermore, regarding breast cancer, the Women's Health Initiative (WHI), which used a synthetic progestin, medroxyprogesterone acetate (MPA), actually increased the risk for breast cancer.[8] In fact, the Nurses' Health Study followed a group of women for 16 years and showed that the addition of synthetic progestin to estrogen resulted in a tripling of the risk for breast cancer![9]

In 2000, a traditional mainline medical journal called the Journal of the National Cancer Institute noted that synthetic progestins increase breast cancer by approximately 25 percent.[10] Yet, ten years later, I still notice doctors out there, still writing prescriptions for synthetic progestins.

Meanwhile, in a Danish Study of approximately 80,000 women they showed that the use of synthetic progestins increases the risk of breast cancer.[11] And in a Swedish study, progestins have also shown an increase in the risk for breast cancer.[12]

"Dr. Lee doesn't settle for mediocre,
he aims for perfection."

I had first visited Dr. Lee in 2009 at age 64. Prior to that time, I considered myself in excellent health. I had always gotten a lot of exercise, ran five miles five days a week, ate properly, got plenty of sleep and took a lot of vitamin supplements.

But around late 2008, I began having problems. I was not able to run more than two miles a day and had to walk most of that. I had problems breathing and no longer seemed to have any stamina or strength in my muscles. I couldn't do anything physical (such as yard work or housecleaning) for more than 15-20 minutes without having to sit down and rest. I was feeing extreme fatigue, both mental & physical, problems sleeping, weight gain, mild depression and mood swings.

Dr. Lee spent a couple of hours with me during that first visit and performed several tests to determine the cause of my issues. He changed some of my supplements and added several new ones, took me off the synthetic hormones I had been taking for the past 20 years and started me on bioidentical hormones. The improvements started almost immediately. Progesterone deficiency was one of my diagnoses.

For the past nine months he has continued to make changes to my diet, supplements and hormones—and the improvements have continued. On my first visit, he asked me to rate my energy level. I gave it a two or less on a scale of one to ten. Now, I rate my energy level at eight or higher. I feel a tremendous increase in my energy levels, mental focus and my all over muscle tone has improved. I am not having any problems sleeping, my running is back to normal, I have joined the local gym and go four or five days a week. I feel like I'm 30 again!

Dr. Lee doesn't settle for mediocre, he aims for perfection and he won't stop until he feels there is no more room for improvement.

— Sherry Zellers

Additional Benefits of Bioidentical Progesterone

As for studies that show bioidentical progesterone is beneficial, there are many trials that do indicate a difference. Although evidence-based medicine prefers a randomized controlled study, there are large-scale observational trials and randomized placebo-control primate trials that are readily available. Evidence-based medicine cannot ignore these studies for very much longer.

In 2007, Dr. Agnès Fournier studied over 80,000 postmenopausal women who were all on estrogen. Half the group took bioidentical progesterone and the other half took synthetic progestin. The synthetic progestin group had a higher rate of breast cancer.[13] In a primate study, the use of synthetic progestins led to an increase in marker Ki-67 for breast cancer, whereas bioidentical progesterone did not show an increase in Ki-67.[14]

Low progesterone levels have been shown to indicate lower survival rates for breast cancer when compared to more optimal progesterone levels.[15-16] In another study, progesterone levels had an inverse relationship to breast cancer risk. The higher progesterone had the lowest risk, whereas the lower progesterone had the highest risk for breast cancer.[17] So the question is, at what progesterone level do you want to be?

When the Women's Health Initiative (WHI) study came out in 2002, I remember the intense hype the media created about hormone replacement therapy being associated with a higher risk of breast cancer, heart disease and stroke.

What the media failed to mention was that it was synthetic hormone replacement therapy with Premarin® (horse estrogen) and Provera® (synthetic progesterone). Albeit, this came at a time when the standard medical care for postmenopausal women was the use of Premarin® and Provera® to help prevent breast cancer, heart disease and osteoporosis.

Unfortunately, as well, the media failed to report on the other major study that came out at the same time—a French study, which used bioidentical hormones for almost nine years without any indication for breast cancer from bioidentical hormones.[18] Even more regrettably, the confusion that the media created over the 2002 WHI study—between synthetic hormones and bioidentical hormones—continues to this day.

In regard to heart disease and stroke, synthetic progestin has been shown to increase the risk, whereas progesterone has been shown to reduce the risk. In the WHI study the use of synthetic progestin increased the risk for heart disease and stroke.[19]

Furthermore, there are many studies in which progesterone actually lowers the risks of heart disease and stroke—while augmenting the protective effect of estrogen.[20-22]

Synthetic progestin has been shown to lower HDL (good cholesterol), whereas bioidentical progesterone has been shown to have the desirable effect of raising the good cholesterol.[23] The use of progesterone has been shown to reduce the vasospasm of the coronary artery whereas synthetic progestin can increase vasospasm, which then increases the risk for heart disease and stroke.[24]

Progesterone has been shown to prevent atherosclerotic plaques in the coronary arteries, whereas synthetic progestins did not provide any such beneficial effect.[25-27] Progesterone has also been shown to reduce inflammation and cytokine VCAM (bad blood marker), whereas synthetic progestin has had no such effect.[28]

One of the most amazing effects of bioidentical progesterone is that it helps the brain. In fact, progesterone has been used successfully in clinical trials for people with traumatic brain injury. When I did one of my fellowships at the University of Pittsburgh, there were many clinical trials to determine if there was any special medication, anti-inflammatory agent or cytokine blocker that would help with the survival—and with the recovery—of brain function. All the trials done at the University of Pittsburgh while I was there did not have any positive results. Actually, in the last 20 years, all the large trials to help patients with severe brain injury have all failed.

However, there is now research showing that progesterone helps people with traumatic brain injury. In a 2012 review of the three randomized clinical trials of progesterone for acute traumatic brain injury, it was shown that progesterone improved the neurologic outcome, but also mentioned that more studies are needed.[29]

Another exciting recent clinical trial used progesterone and vitamin D in patients with traumatic brain injury. The study compared a placebo group with a group that received progesterone 1 mg/kg injection intramuscularly (IM) every 12 hours for five days, and Vitamin D 5 micrograms/kg (IM) once a day for five days. The group that received both progesterone and vitamin D had a better outcome, and less of a mortality rate, when compared to the placebo group. It is now believed that both progesterone and vitamin D reduced the brain inflammation.[30]

Progesterone is neuroprotective, which is exactly what you want in order to have a better memory. In the Women's Health Initiative study (WHI), it was noted that postmenopausal women who took the synthetic hormones (Premarin® and Provera®) experienced more dementia, and more cognitive impairment.[31-32]

If bioidentical progesterone helps with your brain, and synthetic progesterone causes memory loss, then which one would you like to take?

Sounds simple, but believe it or not, I just saw a patient of mine who came back from a top university Mayo Clinic... where she was put on Premarin® (horse estrogen) and Provera® (synthetic progesterone). All I could say to her was, "Where do I start?"

"He is there to keep you on track and direct you like a master conductor."

My goal is to age gracefully. This is what brought me to Dr. Lee. I wanted guidance on overcoming some of the things going on in my life which I attributed to aging. I felt tired, had problems sleeping, gained weight, had low energy and just couldn't seem to keep a good exercise routine going.

Dr. Lee listened carefully, asked me many questions, and then went through a PowerPoint presentation explaining why he thought I may need progesterone. Testing confirmed his analysis. Then he helped me understand the cause and effect roles that my hormones play. What I learned is that my body was not balanced, not in tune.

My progesterone is now balanced and I sleep wonderfully, but Dr. Lee did not stop there. He provided wonderful guidance for my weight loss, increased energy and exercise regimen. Most impressive was his use of advanced testing and technology in fine-tuning my personal needs. He teaches what you need to do. Then, as you are performing, he is there to keep you on track and direct you like a master conductor.

— Brigitte Goersch

Progesterone Preferences

The FDA has approved only two bioidentical progesterones — Crinone® vaginal gel and Prometrium® pills. Although my first choice would be to prescribe bioidentical progesterone that is sublingual and made by a reputable compound pharmacist, I have used Prometrium® with favorable results. However, I should explain that taking Prometrium® by mouth exposes the progesterone to extensive changes as it passes through stomach acid, and then the liver, before going into the circulation.

So, to avoid such exposure, my preferred routes of delivery are transdermally or sublingually (under the tongue) for faster absorption. Once a patient is taking progesterone, I've received positive feedback about relief from headaches, anxiety, mood swings, acne, hot flashes, low libido, insomnia and more.

Progesterone Replacement Protecting DNA

The most important structure of your body is your DNA. Every cell in your body has DNA, except your red blood cells. The ends, or caps of your DNA, are called telomeres, and they are the protective parts of your DNA. As you age, your telomeres actually shorten, and there is a critical point when your telomeres shorten to the tipping point. At this tipping point , if there are excessive free radicals or oxidative damage to the cell, the telomeres can no longer protect the DNA. This is when DNA damage will begin. At this time, you will see premature aging, chronic disease, cancer and early death due to DNA damage. Long story short... telomere length has been correlated with the aging process.[33-34]

In a study of 130 postmenopausal women, half the group received hormonal therapy with estrogen and progesterone. The study showed that the women who received hormonal therapy for more than five years had significantly longer telomere lengths when compared to women who did not receive hormonal therapy. This study showed that hormonal therapy slowed down the aging process.[35]

"Now, I sleep like a baby."

I am a 48-year-old woman that was suffering from poor sleep and waking up three or four times in the middle of the night. Before I saw Dr. Lee, my energy was very low and I would wake up exhausted. I'd had a hysterectomy in 2007 due to a large fibroid, and since that time I went into a surgical menopause.

After doing my saliva test, Dr. Lee started me on bioidentical progesterone under the tongue and my sleep improved within four days. Now, I sleep like a baby, my energy is much better and I wake up refreshed.

— Maria Cubelo-Hinton

CHAPTER 5 REVIEW

— Progesterone deficiency starts before estrogen deficiency, and usually presents itself around the age of 35 with: irregular periods, insomnia, irritability, weight gain, tiredness, low libido and hot
flashes.

— Bioidentical progesterone can help protect women from developing
breast cancer, whereas synthetic progesterone increases the risk for
breast cancer.

— For women undergoing hysterectomy, bioidentical progesterone
helps prevent fibroids and/or endometriosis.

— Provera® is a synthetic progesterone that has been associated with
higher rates of breast cancer, heart disease, stroke and blood clots. I
strongly advise against the use of Provera®.

— Bioidentical progesterone reduces inflammation. Synthetic progesterone does not.

— The FDA has approved only two bioidentical progesterones—Cri-
none® vaginal gel and Prometrium® pills. Although my first choice
would be to prescribe bioidentical progesterone that is sublingual
and made by a reputable compound pharmacist, I have used Pro-
metrium® with favorable results.

6

TESTOSTERONE

**It's time to dispel the prostate cancer myth,
once and for all.**

Not just women are subject to hormonal imbalance. For my male patients that are complaining of tiredness, I usually discover they have a low testosterone level, or they are in a condition called andropause. Andropause is when a man's testosterone level is in decline. It's similar to a woman going into menopause and experiencing a decline in estrogen, except that andropause is a decline in testosterone. Symptoms of andropause consist of fatigue, low libido, decrease in physical fitness, loss of muscle mass, loss of bone density, lack in competitive drive and erectile dysfunction.

Although andropause can cause some of the above symptoms, they usually don't present as acutely as the symptoms women experience in menopause. In fact, most men that are going through andropause are not even aware of it, and usually accept that their tiredness is part of the aging process. Then, after the adjustments of andropause, testosterone levels continue to decline as men age.[1] In fact, after approximately the age of 25, a man's testosterone level begins to decrease and will continue to gradually decline for the rest of his life.[2]

Unfortunately, andropause is a lethal condition that's associated with diabetes, cancer, heart disease, stroke, memory loss, Alzheimer's and early mortality. Low testosterone is associated with aging of the cardiovascular system and the brain. It's also associated with an elevation of chronic inflammation. Remember, chronic inflammation accelerates the aging process and is the gateway to chronic disease. Markers for inflammations include the cytokines of interleukin-6 and tumor necrosis factor alpha.

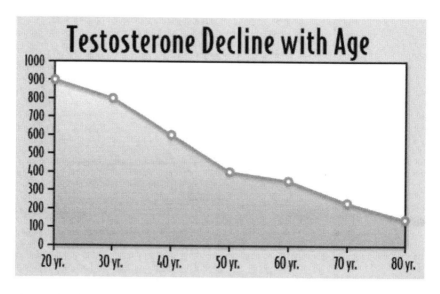

As serum testosterone levels progressively decline with age for men, the resulting pathophysiological changes are typically a lower sex drive and declining energy levels.

Fortunately, testosterone replacement therapy has been shown to reduce the inflammation markers of interleukin-6 and tumor necrosis factor alpha.[3] However, the treatment of andropause in conventional medicine is not yet widely accepted—unless you have a level lower than the reference range. I really believe if you wait that long before starting treatment, then you've already missed the boat for making significant improvements.

"Believe me, andropause does happen—
we just don't want to admit it's happening to us."

When I turned 50 I seemed to hit a wall. I've been active all my life—lifting weights and working out religiously for the past 20 years—but suddenly, I was losing strength along with my drive. I felt tired and run-down every day, and was starting to get depressed, which was something I had never felt before. Something was wrong and I needed help.

Based on a strong recommendation, I went to see Dr. Lee in February 2010. We talked extensively about what I was going through. He was very caring and concerned about my situation. He immediately put me through an extensive panel of blood work to determine what could be causing my problems. We discovered that my testosterone was very low and my body was no longer producing testosterone on its own. Dr. Lee diagnosed me with andropause and hypogonadism.

We discussed my options, along with the amount of research that has been done regarding testosterone replacement therapy. I felt very comfortable with the information and made the decision to proceed. We started therapy with a compounded testosterone gel, which seemed to work for the first couple of months. I began to feel a little better and my energy increased, but it seemed to be short-lived as my "good feelings" began to drop back to the levels I experienced before. So I made the call to Dr. Lee, who was quick to respond with a switch to testosterone injections. Dr. Lee is so easy to talk with about anything—you always feel relaxed and confident that he is on your team.

Now, after being on the injections for a few months, I feel like I'm reliving my 30s again! I have so much more energy and am actually making strength gains in the gym again—even at 51! I know there have been doubts about men having andropause; but believe me, andropause does happen—we just don't want to admit it's happening to us.

I have to thank Dr. Lee for giving me back my life, and for helping me get through this very difficult time. I really do not know of many doctors whose main concern is to truly help you be the best person you can be. My depression is gone, and I can honestly say every day is better and better.

— Bryan Bailey

As for testosterone and its relationship with coronary artery disease, there are some small clinical numbers showing that testosterone replacement has reduced angina attacks and ischemic episodes.[4-5]

A 2012 study showed that testosterone replacement in 1,031 men (over 40 years, with a serum testosterone under 250 ng/dl) had a lower rate of death compared to the group that did not receive testosterone. Thus, the study further supports the importance of the use of testosterone in men.[6]

A review of testosterone and coronary artery disease in the aging male shows that the aging male has lower testosterone, increased mediators (or markers) for atherosclerosis and that...

...replacement therapy with testosterone has reduced atherosclerosis.

It is important to have your blood count monitored while on testosterone replacement because testosterone can cause polycythemia, which is an elevated red blood cell count that can thicken the blood and cause stroke or clotting.

Are You Anabolic or Catabolic?

Because testosterone is an anabolic hormone, it can help increase protein synthesis—thereby improving your body's ability to build muscle and lose fat. This is important because, with aging, a condition may occur in which the body sacrifices muscle in order to provide energy. This is a catabolic condition. Fortunately, there is a 24-hour urine test by Genova Diagnostics® that will determine if you are in an anabolic condition (where you are building up muscle) or in a catabolic condition (where you are losing muscle).

If you are losing muscle, testosterone therapy can help you go from catabolic to anabolic. In addition, testosterone replacement for women has been shown to improve on low bone mass.[7] For this reason, I often offer small doses of testosterone to my female patients—once they are balanced with estrogen and progesterone.

Libido

Testosterone can also help improve libido—for men and women. Women will need to have their estrogen and progesterone balanced first; however, before trying to optimize testosterone levels in women, I always explain that their low libido is one of the most challenging things to treat with hormonal therapy. In fact, I have seen some female patients with testosterone levels higher than some male patients, yet those women still have a low libido.

Typically, men that complain of low libido also say they no longer have a morning erection, or are experiencing erectile dysfunction. (Generally, such information is not volunteered freely by men; but, when asked directly, most will answer honestly!)

Also, by the time a male patient usually sees me for their low libido or erectile dysfunction, they've already been prescribed the blue pill (Viagra®). Which is why the first thing I normally do after optimizing their testosterone is to take them off the blue pill so... they can test it out for a few days. Then, if their erectile dysfunction has not significantly improved, I will place them on Viagra®, Cialis® or Levitra®.

At that point, should the testosterone and the pharmacologic remedies not prove helpful, then the next steps include: injections into the penis; a vacuum tumescence pump (penis pump); or—the option that seems to give a lot of men the most satisfaction with their erectile dysfunction—a penile implant performed by their urologist.

However, even once corrected, erectile dysfunction is still a sign of poor circulation (chronic inflammation) and an indicator of early heart disease. In fact, it was recently estimated that men experiencing the onset of erectile dysfunction may very well have a heart attack within three to five years.[8]

"I've been given a fresh, healthy life at 40."

At 39, I considered myself to be in great shape with a very active lifestyle and a consistent routine of running, working out four times a week with a personal trainer, playing in team sports and following a diet I thought to be healthy.

However, I had noticed over the last couple of years that I was slowly gaining weight and losing some of my "youthful energy." I didn't pay much attention to the changes and just attributed them to getting older. But then, in November 2009, I was at our family doctor for a routine checkup and happened to read an article about low testosterone. I asked my doctor about it and she said we could do a blood test.

When I went back in two weeks for the results, I was told that my counts were a little low, but my doctor "thought" they were still within normal range. I questioned her about what the level was supposed to be, but she couldn't give me a confident response.

Because of that unsure response, my wife researched low testosterone on the Internet and urged me to see an endocrinologist. Having recently read a magazine article about Dr. Edwin Lee, she called and scheduled my appointment.

I first saw Dr. Lee in January 2010. I liked him the minute I met him. He diagnosed my symptoms, and then explained how my symptoms were affecting my daily routine and overall health. He asked what my goals were—my personal and physical goals, as well as my overall health goals—and then explained how we could achieve those goals.

As soon as my test results came back and confirmed I had low testosterone, Dr. Lee started treatment to bring my levels up. After a couple of weeks, I started to feel more energy throughout the day, more motivated to push myself even more in the gym and at work, and my overall general health was improving. My wife really took notice of my increase in my energy, as well as my libido, and said I wasn't as moody as I had been lately.

I never feel like Dr. Lee is simply giving me a prescription; rather, he gives me a detailed road map to my overall health. I have been seeing Dr. Lee for nine months and I've already achieved my physical goals for which I've been striving most of my life—but could never attain. I have never felt healthier than I do right now. I don't succumb to illness like before, and I am finally getting a good night's sleep. Also, my family life has never been better, which I attribute to my improved mood and overall health.

I have never believed in a "magic pill" or shortcut to anything. The only reason I am sharing my experiences now is that I've been given a fresh, healthy life at 40. I believe in Dr. Lee because he not only corrected the problems I've been having (for who knows how long), but he actually takes interest in my life and goals, and explains how to take advantage of my new health. I have now referred six people to Dr. Lee—and they're becoming believers as well.

I hope that anyone who questions the way they feel, and desires to perform better, will take Dr. Lee's advice and change their life.

— *Dave Kreutzer*

Testosterone Conversion

Testosterone can either be converted into estrogen (estradiol) by an enzyme called aromatase, or it can be converted into dihydrotestosterone (DHT) by an enzyme called 5-alpha reductase. Throughout life, your body requires certain levels of estradiol and DHT. For example, if a male child is born with a deficiency of 5-alpha reductase, he will have underdeveloped male genitalia and a small prostate. Often, these boys are raised as girls due to their underdeveloped genitalia.

At the other end of the spectrum, there is data showing that benign prostate hypertrophy is related to high levels of DHT. Although the prostate cancer link with DHT and estradiol levels is still undecided, with data supporting both sides,[9-10] I believe in proactively preventing high DHT levels through the use of saw palmetto and/or a 5-alpha reductase inhibitor, such as finasteride.[11]

As for my overweight male patients with low testosterone, they almost always have high estradiol levels; which lead to, among other things, man boobs—that usually go away when their estradiol levels are reduced. To reduce their estradiol levels, I often use a low dose of anastrazole to inhibit the aromatase enzyme that converts testosterone into estradiol.

Usually, when they lose enough weight, I will discontinue their use of anastrazole. Or, occasionally, I will prescribe a low dose of tamoxifen to maintain their estradiol levels. In the next section of this chapter, I will address the myth of testosterone and prostate cancer; however, I do believe the real concern should be more about this type of aromatase activity (high estrogen with low testosterone) and its association with prostate cancer.[12]

The Prostate Cancer Myth

This brings us to another controversial issue in medicine. Many doctors have been trained to believe that giving testosterone can increase the risk of prostate cancer (due to an elevation of the prostate-specific antigen) on the basis of one article in 1941 by Dr. Charles B. Huggins in which one of three men with prostate cancer was treated with testosterone.

Dr. Huggins reported that one man's testosterone treatment caused an elevation of a blood test called acid phosphatase, and then he concluded that testosterone can cause prostate cancer. The blood test acid phosphatase has since been abandoned, and there are now better markers for prostate cancer.[13]

Conversely, in a recent study of men with low testosterone, restoring their testosterone to normal levels has not been associated with an increased incidence of prostate cancer. Also, to date there is absolutely no data supporting the theory that restoring testosterone increases prostate cancer.[14]

Furthermore, there is evidence that men undergoing treatment for prostate cancer, and being treated with testosterone, show no increase in recurrence of prostate cancer.[15] Thus, Dr. Huggins' 1941 myth that testosterone can cause prostate cancer is not clinically supported.

Overall goals for total testosterone for a male are 600 ng/dL or higher. For women, above 40 ng/dL. For bioavailable testosterone, the goals are 500 or higher in men, and above 20 for women. Polycythemia, elevated hemoglobin and liver function tests will need to be monitored on a regular basis. Men will also need a prostate-specific antigen (PSA) test on a regular basis. Side effects—especially for women—can be acne, deepening of the voice or unwanted hair.

"I went to Dr. Lee seeking a fountain of youth, and I wasn't disappointed."

Eighteen years ago, I built my own softball "field of dreams" in Kentucky. But a few years ago, the younger players in my tournaments began hitting too many home runs, so I moved the outfield fence further back. Unfortunately, though, I couldn't hit any more home runs—and at 67, I still love to play softball! I also noticed that I was losing muscle, gaining weight and losing some strength in my workouts.

I went to Dr. Lee seeking a fountain of youth, and I wasn't disappointed. He balanced my hormones with supplements, treated me for lead and mercury toxicity, and helped me correct my eating habits. My testosterone is now where it should be and I feel strong again. My thrill this summer was hitting four home runs. I can't wait until my first game next year!

— *Mike Borders*

One case that I would like to share occurred when a male physician was seeing me about his constant tiredness, loss of libido and weight gain. During his work-up, he noted that he used to have a lot of energy, but over the course of several years his energy level had slowly been decreasing. In addition, he noted that he had gained some weight or belly fat, and it was hard for him to lose it. His testosterone was very low and he was noted to have early bone loss. Rather than just using testosterone, I had him do a special test to see if his pituitary gland (in the middle of the brain) was functioning properly, and it was. Then, with testosterone therapy underway, he soon started reversing his tiredness and regained his energy.

However, replacing testosterone in male patients is not always that easy. My male patients using testosterone in a cream or a gel are often the ones who achieve optimal results—but, this may not be the ideal way to do so if one has a pituitary gland problem which is causing low testosterone. I see many men who suffered multiple head traumas (car accidents, sports related injuries or falls) many years ago which, years later, resulted in low testosterone. It is crucial to identify the root cause of low testosterone. If the cause of low testosterone is from the pituitary, then one may benefit from certain medications, like Clomid® or HCG (human chorionic gonadotropin), that help you produce your own testosterone naturally.

"My primary physician had diagnosed me with low testosterone, but was having trouble bringing it back to a healthy level."

After being in good health throughout my life, I began experiencing some general aches and pains, poor recovery from exercise and increased fatigue.

I'm a psychologist and that means I'm sitting for several hours a day. In addition, I'd recently turned 40 and so I figured that the onset of middle age, combined with sitting at work all day, was negatively impacting my overall physical well-being. My primary physician had diagnosed me with low testosterone, but was having trouble bringing it back to a healthy level.

After seeing a magazine article about Dr. Lee, and reading that he'd been the team endocrinologist for the Cleveland Indians (I'm a baseball fan!), I decided to set up an appointment. On our first session, he conducted a thorough history of my symptoms and spent a great deal of time listening to my concerns. He set up a plan for some blood work and, upon receiving the results, recommended testosterone injections and vitamin D supplementation.

Now, after a year of working with Dr. Lee, my testosterone and vitamin D are consistently at optimal levels, my energy has increased greatly, my stamina has improved and my aches have reduced markedly!

— Richard Marcil

Another way to help increase the level of testosterone is with the use of pregnenolone with DHEA substrates that convert into testosterone. If the cause is from testicular failure, then the treatment will most likely be testosterone replacement—whether it is used under the tongue, transdermally (gels, creams, patches) or by injections.

I would not recommend the use of testosterone by mouth since there have been many negative side effects noted in medical literature. For most of my women patients, I have them on either a small dose of a gel, cream or under the tongue. As always, it is crucial to monitor for any side effects.

"I felt as if my joints were being bathed
in a nourishing fluid."

Just three to four hours after my first testosterone application, I felt as if my joints were being bathed in a nourishing fluid. My chest cavity opened up, my shoulders went back and I stood as straight as if I was 30 years old. I was unprepared for this and I remember thinking, "Now I know what a dry plant must feel like when it has finally been watered."

— William Cameron
Former Canadian bobsled team member

Testosterone Therapy for Women

For women, testosterone levels may start dropping about ten years before menopause. Then, after the onset of menopause, most women have very low testosterone levels. By the way, testosterone in women comes from the ovaries—from the conversion of the adrenal sex hormone, DHEA. Usually I hear that their libido has disappeared, or they tell me their husband is requesting that I help improve on this condition. Besides a low sex drive, many of them also need help with their weight. It is very difficult for women to lose weight when they do not have enough of their anabolic hormone. In addition, testosterone can help with memory and cognition.

Regarding low libido, a study published in the New England Journal of Medicine has shown that using testosterone helped women with a low libido. This study was done in postmenopausal women—using up to a 300 micrograms patch of testosterone, and no estrogen.[16]

In a study in older women, it was noted that women with higher serum testosterone levels had stronger bones. Testosterone replacement can help women with bone loss, or osteoporosis.[17-18]

Testosterone (administered any way other than swallowing) will improve on lowering cholesterol, and on lowering bad cholesterol, or LDL (desired effect).[19]

In a 2012 study, it was noted that testosterone therapy should become an integral part of hormone therapy in selected postmenopausal women in the future.[20]

Significantly, in a study I think is very impressive, it was found that testosterone inhibits the breast cell proliferation in postmenopausal women. It was a randomized, double-blind, placebo-controlled study (the gold standard of research) in which a group of women received 300 micrograms of testosterone via a patch with estradiol and norethisterone acetate (synthetic progesterone). A sample of the breast was ascertained, and it showed that testosterone protected the breast cells from the stimulation of the estrogen—and from the synthetic progesterone (desired effect).[21]

In a 2013 article entitled, "Testosterone therapy in women: Myths and Misconceptions," it states that testosterone is breast protective. Although promising, I think more studies are needed in this area.[22]

If you are pregnant, testosterone should never ever be used because it can effect the fetus' sexual development. If the fetus is a female, then it may develop male traits due to the testosterone exposure during pregnancy. As with men, testosterone levels must be monitored, in addition to liver function tests and blood counts for polycythemia (elevated red blood cell count).

In one reported case, a woman abused injections of testosterone and developed polycythemia, causing her to have a heart attack. I also advise never taking testosterone by swallowing because it can affect the liver, and cause an increase in cholesterol levels. The most common side effect for women using testosterone may be mild acne, and rare instances of excessive unwanted hair growth. Usually, a woman will get acne before the hair growth.[23]

Testosterone replacement in women can vary. I try not to use testosterone cream in men or in women that have small children at home because of accidentally exposing the children to testosterone, thereby affecting their sexual development. I use a lot of sublingual testosterone in women. I have tried the patch (which can be bulky), with minimal success. Also, on occasion, I have used injections of low-dose testosterone. The use of DHEA can also increase testosterone, but not all the time. Another possible therapy is implantable testosterone.

Testosterone Replacement Protecting DNA

The most important structure of your body is your DNA. Every cell in your body has DNA, except your red blood cells. The ends, or caps of your DNA, are called telomeres, and they are the protective parts of your DNA. As you age, your telomeres actually shorten, and there is a critical point when your telomeres shorten to the tipping point. At this tipping point , if there are excessive free radicals or oxidative damage to the cell, the telomeres can no longer protect the DNA. This is when DNA damage will begin. At this time, you will see premature aging, chronic disease, cancer and early death due to DNA damage. Long story short... telomere length has been correlated with the aging process.[24-25]

The one published study that looks most promising was done in mice. It was a unique study since these were special mice that had no androgen (testosterone) receptors. It was shown in this study that testosterone replacement actually improved in increasing telomere lengths (desired effect) of the heart muscle cells. The conclusion of this study showed that testosterone replacement slowed down the aging process.[26]

More medical studies are needed to see if testosterone replacement can improve on keeping the telomeres healthy, or even increasing their length. I expect that it will.

CHAPTER 6 REVIEW

— Testosterone starts to decline around the age of 25, and continuously decline from that point.

— Low testosterone in men and women presents itself with: fatigue, low libido, decreased bone mass, low bone density, loss of competitive drive and erectile dysfunction (men only).

— Low testosterone in men is a lethal disease and is associated with: diabetes, cancer, heart disease, strokes, memory loss, Alzheimer's and early death.

— For my female patients with low testosterone, I believe you should always balance your estrogen and progesterone first. A goal is to get a total testosterone level above 40 ng/dL or a Free Testosterone level in the top one-third of the reference range.

— For my female patients, never use testosterone if you are pregnant.

— For my male patients over 40 years of age, my goal is to achieve a total testosterone level above 600 mg/dL, while always monitoring for any side effects.

— Men need to have a prostate-specific antigen (PSA) test on a regular basis.

— Testosterone replacement does not cause prostate cancer.

— Testosterone replacement therapy in men and women is important and can be achieved by gel, creams, sublinguals, injections or with DHEA. For men with a pituitary problem, you may need Clomid® or HCG. Testosterone replacement needs to be monitored for any side effects.

7

DHEA

Men with higher levels of DHEA-S
live the longest.

The hormone DHEA (dehydroepiandrosterone) is produced in the adrenals and the brain. As we age, DHEA levels decline. DHEA-S (dehydroepiandrosterone sulfate) is the sulfated version of DHEA. DHEA peak secretion is in the morning and then varies throughout the day; however, DHEA-S has fewer variations and is therefore the preferred hormone to monitor via the blood.

The majority of your DHEA comes from your adrenal glands. As you age, DHEA levels decrease after the age of 20. DHEA levels also decrease with adrenal fatigue, since the adrenal glands secrete the sugar (cortisol), salt (aldosterone) and sex (DHEA) hormones. To see the progression of DHEA levels during adrenal fatigue, please refer to the chart on the next page.[1-2]

"I can't imagine doing without Dr. Lee's guidance and methods."

Once I reached my seventies, I started experiencing a noticeable physical slowdown, weight gain, crankiness and the typical aches and pains that come with age. I was gradually losing interest in many of the things dear to me. My wife (a physician) noticed the change in me, and while regularly checking my pulse, diagnosed me as being in atrial fibrillation.

A visit to the cardiologist confirmed that I was in A-fib, and I was put on heart medication in the hope I would return to normal. It was at this time that I was advised by a colleague to make an appointment with Dr. Lee and get some blood work done—and to especially have my testosterone level checked. The results showed that my testosterone and DHEA levels were extremely low but could be restored to a normal level with periodic injections.

I followed Dr. Lee's advice and the results were almost immediate. Within days, my aches and pains diminished and my energy level rose. In short, I was feeling more normal and alive again. In addition, Dr. Lee prescribed a regimen of vitamin supplements, DHEA and nutrients which were reinforced by a special battery of tests and an exercise plan that greatly improved my general well-being, my home life and my overall outlook on things. Not only was I physically feeling better, but I enjoyed a psychological improvement as well.

Looking back now, I can't imagine doing without Dr. Lee's guidance and methods—which have produced such positive results in such a short time, and which have given me a new lease on life.

— Thomas O'Halloran

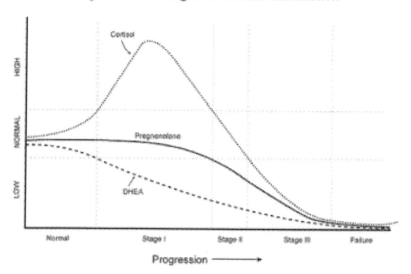

Patterns of salivary cortisol, pregnenolone and DHEA levels in adrenal fatigue.

The DHEA Debacle

The controversy with dehydroepiandrosterone (DHEA) developed in the athletic world, where it is forbidden in many professional sports such as the National Football League, National Basketball Association, Professional Golfers' Association and Professional Cycling. However, there is one professional sport that currently allows the use of DHEA, and that is Major League Baseball.

Even our lawmakers have been involved with DHEA. The Food and Drug Administration first banned the substance in 1985. However, under the Dietary Supplement Health and Education Act nine years later, DHEA not only became legal, it was reclassified as a supplement. In 2004, lawmakers tried to add it to the list of drugs (under the Anabolic Steroid Control Act) that are illegal to obtain without a prescription.

In endocrinology the debate continues over whether DHEA works or not. Even the Mayo Clinic website states that the evidence for DHEA claims is lacking.[3] Low levels of DHEA-S have been associated with obesity, type 2 diabetes, cancer, hypertension, cardiovascular disease, depression, low libido and osteoporosis.[4]

From the Division of Endocrinology, a New England Journal of Medicine article showed that DHEA did not help in elderly men or women. In a two-year placebo-controlled, randomized, double-blind study, DHEA did not show any benefits in body composition, physical performance, insulin sensitivity or quality or life.[5] However, in that study, the use of DHEA was suboptimal.

DHEA Benefits

An earlier, smaller study (also a placebo-controlled, randomized, double-blind study) showed that with 100 mg of DHEA, fat body mass decreased and knee muscle strength and lumbar back strength increased.[6] In another double-blind, placebo-controlled study, 280 elderly men and women were studied to determine if DHEA slowed the aging process. In women, the DHEA increased testosterone, estradiol and also improved the libido, skin and bone turnover.[7]

In a prospective study (a study in which the subjects are identified and then followed forward in time) a 27-year follow-up with men showed in 2008 that low levels of DHEA-S predict a higher risk for early mortality. The study showed that men with higher levels of DHEA-S (> 200 ug/dL) live the longest, while men with lower levels of DHEA-S had higher blood pressure and higher fasting blood sugars, as well as the mortality associated with those conditions.[8]

Furthermore, a New England Journal Medicine article showed that DHEA administered to women with adrenal insufficiency improved their overall well-being, depression, anxiety and libido.[9] When it comes to improving bone density, DHEA replacement of 50 mg a day has been shown to increase hip bone mineral density (BMD) by raising the estradiol levels.[10] Another, more recent 2009 study showed that DHEA replacement improves spine bone mineral density in women and IGF-1 levels in both sexes.[11-12]

Patients with chronic inflammatory bowel disease have been found to have very low levels of DHEA.[13] Levels of DHEA have also been shown to be low in patients with arthritis and in patients with systemic lupus erythematosus.[14-15] The use of DHEA replacement in patients with systemic lupus erythematosus has improved the IGF-1, lowered HDL cholesterol and improved mental well-being and sexuality.[16]

DHEA is a potent inhibitor of interleukin-6 (IL-6).[17] DHEA has been shown to decrease chronic inflammation, and it lowers IL-6 and TNF.[18] DHEA has also been shown to lower nuclear factor kappa beta, and is therefore considered an anti-inflammatory hormone.[19]

For improving memory, a placebo double-blind crossover study found that DHEA at a dose of 300 mg a day in young adults helped with mood and memory. DHEA has helped in the brain area called the hippocampus—which is the area important for memory.[20] DHEA and DHEA-S are both made in the brain and both DHEA and DHEA-S have been shown to protect the brain by improving neuron growth and acting as an antioxidant.[21]

In a recent 2009 double-blind, randomized, placebo-controlled phase III trial with the use of 25 mg DHEA in young adolescent girls and young women with adrenal insufficiency, DHEA showed a significant improvement in psychological well-being.[22]

In one of the longest DHEA trials (one year), 106 patients with Addison's disease (no cortisol, aldosterone, or DHEA production) were given either 50 mg of DHEA or a placebo pill. It was a gold standard study (randomized, double-blind, controlled trial) and the group that received DHEA had improvement in body composition, improvement of bone density at the femoral neck of the hip, less fatigue, and improved self esteem. Some minor side effects of acne were noted in a few female subjects. Overall, DHEA helped.[23]

DHEA can also help women who struggle with fertility. One study used DHEA three months prior to in vitro fertilization (IVF)—on women who were poor responders to IVF. The study resulted in more eggs after DHEA supplementation.[24]

In another study of 32 women who were poor responders to IVF, DHEA was also given for three months prior to IVF. It was concluded that DHEA may improve IVF outcome in poor responders. I would advise not to take DHEA once you are pregnant.[25]

DHEA has also been shown to help when it comes to improving insulin resistance. In a double-blind, randomized, placebo-controlled cross over trial, men with verified coronary artery disease were treated with DHEA at 150 mg a day. After 40 days, the treatment was shown to have lowered insulin, cholesterol and glucose levels. Thus, the benefits of DHEA are excellent in reducing the risk factors for heart disease.[26] In another study, DHEA was administered at 25 mg a day and, after two weeks, patients showed an improvement in insulin resistance, fasting glucose and also the lowering of C reactive protein.[27]

Low levels of DHEA have even been shown to predict heart disease. In a prospective study (a study in which the subjects are identified and then followed forward in time) a nine-year follow-up on 1,709 men showed that low serum DHEA and DHEA-S predicted heart disease.

Additionally, the same study showed that men with the lowest quartile (<1.6 microg/ml) of DHEA had the highest risk for heart disease.[28]

Another prospective study showed that a low DHEA-S is associated with heart disease.[29]   Although these studies show that low DHEA predicts heart disease, there has not been a large study conducted to look at whether DHEA can reverse heart disease. However, with the data that DHEA replacement can lower insulin resistance and lower chronic inflammation, and knowing that low DHEA predicts heart disease, I strongly believe that DHEA replacement will have a positive effect in protecting against heart disease in the future.

"For 29 years I consistently ran over 1,000 miles per year."

I have been a long distance runner, and for 29 years I consistently ran over 1,000 miles per year. I am soon to be 70 years old and I have run many early morning six-mile runs with Dr. Lee.

My wife had seen Dr. Lee, and she was making great improvements in her overall health. So last year, I decided to see Dr. Lee because of my low energy, and to help with my peak performance—and to be sure I met my goal of running in the Grandfather Mountain Marathon in Boone, North Carolina this year.

My consultation with Dr. Lee proved to be very fruitful. He noted that my testosterone was very low, and that I had several nutritional deficiencies. He helped balance my sluggish system with supplements such as EPA-DHA and with bioidentical DHEA (from a compound pharmacy) which are starting to make a huge difference in my 69-year-old body! My 5K and 10K times are once again coming down, which gives me hope for next year to again make the trip to Boone and run in the over 70 age group—and possibly be the oldest runner to cross the finish line!

— David Zellers

Regarding DHEA and breast cancer, there is no association of DHEA or DHEA-S with breast cancer according to the Nurses' Health Study,[30] which is considered to be the "grandmother" of women's health studies and represents the single largest cohort study of women. In a study of premenopausal women, there was no association found between DHEA and DHEA-S levels and breast cancer risk overall.[31]

While low levels of DHEA are associated with an increased risk of breast and ovarian cancer,[32] there was no association found between DHEA levels and the risk of prostate cancer.[33] The data on DHEA replacement increasing the risk of prostate cancer is still unknown.[34] Therefore, the use of DHEA for men should include monitoring for prostate cancer.

The use of DHEA is still controversial. Although there is much data showing that low levels of DHEA are harmful and that DHEA replacement has helped in smaller studies, DHEA is still a hormone in need of a large study to validate its use.

Hormonal balance is principled on the balancing all the hormones — including the adrenals, thyroid, progesterone, testosterone, estrogen, melatonin and DHEA. As always, one will see a greater response by balancing all the hormones, rather than by balancing only one.

Side effects of DHEA may include acne in women and a lowering of the good cholesterol HDL. Yet, on the other hand, it is important to note that DHEA has not been associated with breast or prostate cancer. Also DHEA improves your lower fasting glucose, insulin resistance and memory. In addition to its other positive effects, DHEA can also improve low libido.

Since DHEA-S levels fall with aging, and DHEA is beneficial in lowering chronic inflammation, improving bone density, reducing anxiety, improving on well-being and elevating IGF-1, I am therefore wholeheartedly in support of the use of DHEA.

"I started feeling low on energy after
pushing myself pretty hard at work."

A few years ago, my wife saw a strong improvement in her energy level and triathlon racing as a result of Dr. Lee's medical treatment. So, having known of Dr. Lee for some time, and then developing his website, I knew exactly who to call when I started feeling low on energy after pushing myself pretty hard at work.

Dr. Lee put me on a special diet, vitamin regimen and hormone treatment for my adrenal fatigue, low DHEA and low testosterone. Within a couple of months I was feeling much better, with much higher energy levels, which have continued to this day. I highly recommend Dr. Lee to friends and family—even my mother, who is 80, now sees him!

— Bill Sands

CHAPTER 7 REVIEW

— DHEA (dehydroepiandrosterone) is a hormone produced in the adrenals and the brain. As you age, your DHEA levels decline.

— DHEA is banned from most professional sports since it is linked to improved athletic performance.

— You can monitor DHEA by saliva testing, or by checking DHEA-S by blood test.

— In a 27-year follow-up study, men with higher DHEA-S (above 200 ug/dL) lived longer when compared to men with lower DHEA-S levels.

— DHEA helps: reduce inflammation, improve memory, improve libido, increase energy and increase IGF-1 (a desirable effect in that it counters the aging process).

— DHEA replacement needs to be monitored for side effects and can be administered orally or, as I prefer, sublingually.

8

GROWTH HORMONE

"The ultimate measure of a man
is not where he stands
in moments of comfort and convenience,
but where he stands
at times of challenge and controversy."
— Martin Luther King, Jr.

Out of all the hormones that are administered, growth hormone is the most controversial. Several magazines, including TIME Magazine, have published many articles on the benefits of growth hormone and how to live to 100 years and beyond. Such information has led to growth hormone being touted as the fountain of youth, while many professional and amateur athletes have been caught using growth hormone for enhancing athletic performance.

Growth hormone is secreted from the pituitary gland in a pulsatile fashion—which means that it can be low one time and high another. The largest peak of growth hormone is during the nighttime about an hour after the onset of sleep. A number of factors affect the secretion of growth hormone, such as exercise, diet, age, hormones and stress.

Stimulators of growth hormone secretions include: sleep, melatonin, intense aerobic exercise, low glucose, the dietary protein arginine and the growth hormone releasing hormone known as ghrelin. Inhibitors of growth hormone secretion include: somatostatin, high dietary carbohydrates, low DHEA-S, obesity, high cortisol and a low thyroid.

Growth hormone is important for growth and increasing height until around 18 to 20 years of age. After that, growth hormone is needed as an adult for cellular repair and healing. Other benefits have included: a decrease in body fat, an increase in muscle mass, an increase in bone density, an increase in energy levels, an improved skin tone and an increase in immune function. In addition, it has become popular for regenerative medicine and weight management.[1]

Since growth hormone is an anabolic agent (for building muscle), human growth hormone (HGH) has been used in sports since the 1970s, and it has been banned by the Olympics and the National Collegiate Athletic Association. Beginning at the 2004 Olympic Games in Athens, blood tests were conducted to detect HGH. These tests were implemented because the previously used urine drug screen could not tell the difference between natural and artificial HGH.[2]

Because growth hormone is secreted in a pulsatile fashion, blood levels of growth hormone will vary throughout the day. Growth hormone goes to the liver and secretes another hormone called insulin-like growth factor-1 (IGF-1). IGF-1 plays an important role for growth in children and for the anabolic effect in adults. I consider IGF-1 to be the active growth hormone. IGF-1 binds to IGF binding protein-3 (the carrier protein for IGF-1) and since IGF-1 does not fluctuate as much, it is an ideal screening test for growth hormone deficiency or excess.

Almost every cell is affected by IGF-1, which is important for regulating cell growth, and is a potent inhibitor of programmed cell death. Growth hormone deficiency, according to researchers, is defined as whenever the IGF-1 value falls below 100 ng/ml; however, most endocrinologists would differ on that value.

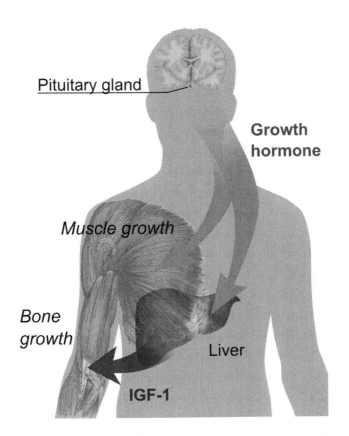

Pituitary gland

Growth hormone

Muscle growth

Bone growth

Liver

IGF-1

Growth hormone being released from the pituitary gland and activating the release of IGF-1 from the liver.

Your peak growth hormone level is around 20 years of age, and by the time you're 30 your growth hormone is already starting to rapidly decrease. Then, as your growth hormone continues to decline, your body gradually loses the ability to repair cell damage, which contributes to aging.

"I struggled with what most people (including some physicians) would classify as classic symptoms of depression."

Prior to being diagnosed by Dr. Lee with a rare condition known as adult-onset GHD (growth hormone deficiency), I struggled with what most people (including some physicians) would classify as classic symptoms of depression. I had a lack of energy, low libido and chronic fatigue. I was also suffering from what seemed like a lack of strength and/or endurance, and I was VERY irritable. I was 5'9" at 225 pounds and was borderline diabetic.

Since Dr. Lee began treatment for my adult-onset GHD, my quality of life and how I feel are unbelievable. I've regained my energy level, libido, strength, endurance and my patience is remarkable. Dr. Lee has been actively working with me to improve my quality of life through a combination of medicine, exercise and nutrition. I run 10 to 15 miles a week and bicycle up to 180 miles, depending on the time of year.

Dr. Lee is always on the cutting edge of what is going on in his field. I recently was going through a tough spot in my training and felt like I was slipping back into a place I did not want to be again. Dr. Lee ordered a simple blood test and found that my body was severely deficient in several areas. Dr. Lee made some adjustments to my treatment through nutritional supplementation, and with a drug to stop my body from converting testosterone to estrogen.

Now I am back to feeling like I am on top of the world. Thank you Dr. Lee for positively effecting not just my life, but also the quality at which I am living it.

— Jason Holland

"All my symptoms have disappeared."

Let me start off by personally thanking Dr. Lee for my newfound health and vitality. For years I had been plagued with chronic fatigue, recurrent infections, pitting edema and excessive weight gain.

Dr. Lee's medical expertise finally led to the discovery that I was suffering from adult-onset GHD (growth hormone deficiency). Since I've started physiologic replacement therapy, all my symptoms have disappeared and I've been able to come off disability to continue my profession as a pediatrician. Kudos to Dr. Lee!

— Raul Alvarez M.D.

Two of the more recognized studies on the effect of age-related changes of IGF-1 concentration across the adult life span come from cross-sectional data collected in two large groups in two different geographical areas: the Baltimore Longitudinal Study of Aging (BLSA) conducted in the United States and the Invecchiare nel CHIANTI (InCHIANTI) study in Italy. The aim of these studies is to verify whether the age-associated decrease in IGF-1 is consistent across different populations and to determine its rate of decline.

The BLSA is an ongoing long-term study of normal human aging conducted by the Intramural Research Program of the National Institute on Aging since 1958 as an open-panel study that continuously recruits volunteers from the Washington–Baltimore area. Total IGF-1 data was available for 604 participants (131 women and 473 men) ranging from 21 to 94 years.

The InCHIANTI study is a large epidemiological study investigating factors affecting mobility in older people. The 1,290 participants were randomly selected from the population of two small towns located in Tuscany, Italy. The current report is based on data from those 559 men and 731 women (ranging in age from 21 to 102 years), with complete data available on total IGF-1.

In the chart on the next page, the IGF-1 data from these two studies were analyzed using linear regression that included study, age, sex and two-way interactions between study, age and sex as independent variables.

In addition, these studies determined that in both men and women: (1) the magnitude of per-year decline in IGF-1 was highest at younger ages and lowest at older ages; (2) the rate of decline was faster in women than in men before the age of 55; (3) the rate of decline was similar in the two sexes at older ages; and (4) in participants older than 50 years, IGF-1 declined with age at a consistent annual rate.

IGF-1 By Age

(Changes in IGF-1 per year from regression modeling)

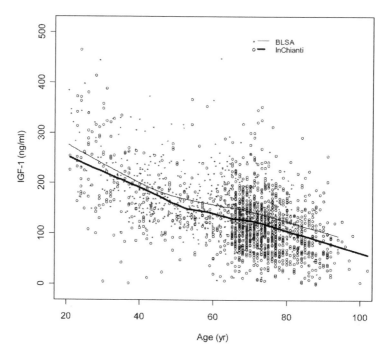

The data for the BLSA and the InCHIANTI studies are reported as scatterplots and summarized by Lowess smoothing curves. The relationship between declining IGF-1 levels and increasing age is clearly illustrated.

(Marcello Maggio, Alessandro Ble, Gian Paolo Ceda and E. Jeffrey Metter. Longitudinal Studies Section Clinical Research Branch National Institute on Aging, National Institutes of Health Baltimore, Maryland; Department of Internal Medicine and Biomedical Sciences Section of Geriatrics, University of Parma, Italy.)

In my private practice, I've discovered adult-onset growth hormone deficiency in many patients that have had some type of head trauma. Some of my patients had suffered from a motor vehicle injury to the head, or a head trauma from a sporting event. It is estimated that 15 percent of head traumas have growth hormone deficiency.[3] Side effects of radiation therapy or head tumors have been shown to effect the production of growth hormone up to ten years later. Also, other hormonal deficiencies can occur after radiation to the brain—like hypothyroidism and adrenocorticotropic hormone (ACTH) deficiency, damage to the pituitary gland (located in the brain) that causes adrenal failure (or cortisol failure).[4-5]

In 1990, a study published in the New England Journal by Dr. Daniel Rudman noted that HGH in men ranging in age from 61 to 81 had significant improvement and reversed the aging process. HGH improved lean body mass, decreased fat, increased bone density and increased skin thickness.[6] Regarding inflammation, growth hormone deficiency has been shown to have higher levels of markers of inflammation, C-reactive protein (CRP), vascular cell adhesion molecule -1 (VCAM-1) and a higher rate of heart disease.[7-8] The use of growth hormone has been shown to lower the markers of inflammation.[9]

HGH Concerns

The controversy over the use of HGH began in 2004 when the federal laws of the United States prohibited the use of HGH—for anything other than the treatment of: short stature due to Turner syndrome, chronic renal failure, Prader-Willi syndrome, idiopathic short stature (ISS) and adult-onset GHD (growth hormone deficiency).

At the beginning of 2007, the federal government made attempts to start enforcing the law on doctors prescribing HGH beyond that narrow range of conditions. It is interesting that lawmakers find it more important to prevent athletes from cheating than it is to keep ordinary adults healthy.

The use of HGH is the ideal way to treat adult-onset growth hormone deficiency, or insufficiency. Because I am a board certified endocrinologist, I have used HGH extensively. I feel comfortable in using HGH; however, I only prescribe it if the patient undergoes a stimulation test and demonstrates that they have adult-onset growth hormone deficiency. There are doctors who prescribe HGH after making a diagnosis with just an IGF-1 level. While an IGF-1 level is a great screening test, it should be followed by a stimulation test—such as an insulin-induced hypoglycemia test to confirm that they have this condition.

There are other growth hormone stimulation tests—such as the arginine test, arginine-GHRH test or glucagon stimulation test—for determining if someone has growth hormone deficiency.[10-11] I prefer the insulin-induced hypoglycemia test since it takes less time, and it is considered the gold standard test in endocrinology.

An insulin-induced hypoglycemia test needs to be done in a doctor's office, or in a hospital setting, due to its many procedures. I have done this test extensively, and learned to do them in my endocrinology fellowship training program at the University of Pittsburgh. An intravenous line is inserted for the injection of insulin—and also for emergency backup in case someone needs to receive intravenous glucose immediately. A baseline glucose and growth hormone is drawn and then fast acting insulin is injected intravenously, depending on the patient's weight and glucose. Then, after the injection of insulin, the blood sugar will drop to a critical point, at which the brain will tell the rest of the body that it needs sugar. At that point ,the glucose may be less than 50 mg/dl and the body is in an emergency mode to help the brain to get more sugar. Glucagon, catecholamine, cortisol and growth hormone are all released to help increase the body's production of glucose or sugar. Once the patient has a reaction to the low glucose (such as: mild tremors, shakes, headache, dizziness, nausea, etc.) and a finger stick glucose check with a glucometer shows a low glucose, then a second glucose and growth hormone is drawn. After that, the last glucose and growth hormone is drawn. Then the patient needs to drink a sugar content drink, like a real soda or orange juice, followed by eating some candy and then a sandwich. Once the finger stick glucose is over 80 and the patient feels fine, then the patient leaves the office.

An insulin-induced hypoglycemia test where the blood glucose is less than 50 mg/dl and the growth hormone does not stimulate above 5 ng/ml is considered to be not normal (the patient has adult-onset growth hormone deficiency). If the growth hormone stimulates over 5 ng/ml then the patient has a normal result and does not have growth hormone deficiency. Since the FDA highly regulates the dispensing of this hormone, it is prudent for the health care provider to confirm that the patient actually has adult-onset growth hormone deficiency. There are doctors who have lost their medical licenses for dispensing human growth hormone because of not performing the growth hormone stimulation test.

Another unfounded controversy is centered around the belief that HGH may cause diabetes or cancer. In a large study called the Pfizer International Metabolic Database (with 40,000 patient years of data on the use of the HGH called Genotropin®), it was established that growth hormone replacement is not associated with an increased risk of new cancer or diabetes—plus, it also showed a dramatic increase in quality of life![12-13] The side effects of HGH are swelling, carpal tunnel syndrome or joint pain. Usually, if you reduce the dose the side effects resolve themselves. There are currently six recombinant growth hormones approved by the FDA: Humatrope®, Genotropin®, Norditropin®, Tev-Tropin®, Saizen® and Nutropin®.

Another difficult issue with using HGH is that the cost can be prohibitive ($300 to $1,500 a month). I've had many patients who qualify for the use of HGH, and then undergo the testing and imaging tests needed, only to have their insurance company reject it. For the short-stature children that are constantly being picked on for their size (resulting in extremely low self-confidence), HGH can have significantly positive results. It breaks my heart when the insurance companies reject the use of it in those situations. That is one of many reasons why I got out of conventional medicine and am no longer dictated to by the insurance companies.

Even though we now know that increasing your IGF-1 levels will slow the manifestations of aging (such as decreasing fat, increasing muscle mass, increasing bone density, strengthening the immune system, improving memory and increasing energy) [14] the FDA does not consider aging as a medical reason for the use of HGH.

However, there are other ways to improve on elevating your IGF-1. The best way is to sleep better, and get at least eight hours of undisturbed sleep. I have many patients whose IGF-1 improves with better sleep. Another way is to exercise by doing high intensity workouts. Also, reducing insulin levels and taking L-Arginine (Amino Acid) will increase your IGF-1.

There is also a very popular herb used in Chinese medicine for arthritis, calcium deficiency and as a growth tonic for children. It's deer or elk velvet antler. There are many companies that sell antler velvet to improve on growth hormone, but I have not seen any clinical data or any published medical literature showing that it can increase IGF-1 or growth hormone levels. There was a study on deer antler velvet looking at IGF-1, muscular strength, red cell mass, testosterone, Vo2 Max (see Chapter 12) and other parameters, and after a ten-week program there was no improvement or change in endocrine (IGF-1, testosterone), red cell mass and Vo2 Max.[15] Another ten-week study looked at female and male rowers, and it also showed no change in IGF-1 levels with elk antler velvet.[16]

Having said this, please be aware that while the Internet has a multitude of products claiming to promote HGH release, most of these products are in fact just expensive scams.

"Like a detective, Dr. Lee thoroughly evaluated
all of my hormone levels."

I was a healthy endurance athlete until I became fatigued all of the time, did not sleep well and woke up every morning exhausted. Every day I felt my healthy life slipping away at only 55. I consulted with many specialists and they were unable to identify why I was feeling so sick. My blood test results were normal. Physically and mentally exhausted, I had almost given up when my primary care physician suggested I see Dr. Lee.

Like a detective, Dr Lee thoroughly evaluated all of my hormone levels and discovered many deficiencies. Then, when I began hormone therapy and started taking growth hormone, my quality of life returned. I sleep better now than I have in many years and do not feel fatigued all of the time. I will be running a marathon in three weeks and then plan on training and completing my first half Ironman Triathlon this fall. Thank you Dr. Lee for giving me back my healthy life.

— Heather Simpson

Growth Hormone Replacement Protecting DNA

The most important structure of your body is your DNA. Every cell in your body, except for red blood cells, has DNA. The ends, or caps, of your DNA are called telomeres, and they are the protective part of your DNA. As you age, the length of your telomeres will shorten. This shortening process will reach a critical point where your telomeres shorten to the tipping point. At this tipping point, if there are excessive free radicals or oxidative damage to the cell—where the telomeres can no longer protect the DNA—then DNA damage will begin, and you will experience premature aging, chronic disease, cancer and early death due to DNA damage. In other words, telomere length has been correlated with the aging process.[17-18]

Although there are no medical studies that show the use of growth hormone will increase telomere length, there are studies that show how higher IGF-1 is associated with longer telomere lengths. In the beginning of this chapter, I discussed that lower levels of IGF-1 are associated with diminished longevity. In a recent study done with 476 healthy Italians, it was show that the higher IGF-1 levels are associated with longer telomere lengths.[19]

In a study published in the Journal of Clinical Endocrinology and Metabolism, it was shown in a group of 2,744 elderly men that the men with the shortest telomere lengths had the lowest IGF-1 levels, and the group with the longest telomere lengths had the highest IGF-1 levels.[20]

I expect that future studies on human growth hormone replacement will improve on telomere lengths, and thus protect the DNA.

"Getting older is great—right?"

I am a 62-year-old male who has been exercising seriously for 32 years. I used to run 35 miles a week. Now I bicycle 150 miles a week and strength train. In spite of those good habits, I was feeling very tired and sleepy during the day, was irritable, and my libido was declining rapidly.

I heard about Dr. Lee and made an appointment. He spent considerable time with me gathering information, and he had some blood and other tests run. I immediately took to him because he is a serious athlete as well.

Dr. Lee found that I suffered from low testosterone, vitamin D deficiency and possibly growth hormone deficiency. Getting older is great—right?

He immediately prescribed testosterone and several natural supplements. I began to feel better within a couple of weeks. About three months ago, I underwent the necessary tests to determine growth hormone deficiency and, I was in fact, deficient. I have been on HGH for two months now and I feel so much better. My mood greatly improved, and I feel stronger and more energetic.

I am very grateful to Dr. Lee and believe every aging male who just doesn't feel like himself anymore should see this great doctor.

— Dave Richardson

CHAPTER 8 REVIEW

— Growth hormone helps: burn fat, increase muscle mass, increase bone density, improve immune system, increase energy and improve skin tone.

— Insulin-like growth factor-1 (IGF-1) is the preferred way to monitor growth hormone levels. IGF-1 is measured in the blood.

— IGF-1 is the active hormone of growth hormone. A desirable IGF-1 level is above 250 ng/mL.

— Your peak growth hormone level occurs around the age of 20, and begins to continuously decline afterwards.

— As your growth hormone declines, your body loses the ability to repair cell damage, and that contributes to aging.

— Adult-onset growth hormone deficiency can occur after a history of head trauma—even a decade or more after the trauma.

— You should see an endocrinologist that does the proper testing to diagnosis adult-onset growth hormone deficiency. The gold standard test is the insulin-induced hypoglycemia test in which you receive intravenous insulin to make your blood sugar drop, and then your growth hormone response to the low blood sugar is measured.

— The best, but most expensive, treatment that can help improve your growth hormone levels is human growth hormone (while being monitored for any side effects).

9

Nutrition

"More die in the United States of too much food than of too little."
— John Kenneth Galbraith

During my previous practice in endocrinology and diabetes, I was a big believer in the American Diabetes Association (ADA) diet. I truly believed that all diabetics should receive eight hours of ADA education on diabetes—the complications of diabetes, the treatment of diabetes and the diet for a diabetic. I also believed that ADA-approved artificial sweeteners were safe. Now, after years of treating patients for their damaging effects, I am totally against the ADA diet and artificial sweeteners.

After studying the many theories on nutrition, while focusing on what is good and bad for diabetics, I began to realize that the ADA does not discriminate between a complex carbohydrate and a simple carbohydrate. Also, the ADA recommendation of the amount of carbohydrates is much too high for most type 2 diabetics. On the ADA diet, diabetics can eat bread, muffins, cereals, pasta, rice, potatoes and oatmeal; however, it's always amazing to see the dramatic improvement in someone's blood sugars just by reducing these simple carbohydrates in their daily intake.

My usual advice for the first six weeks is to eliminate the white sins —anything with white flour, such as: bread, pasta, oatmeal, cereals, rice and potatoes. And, to increase your fiber intake to two or three servings of vegetables per meal—including breakfast.

"Got Veggies?"

Upon recommending these adjustments in diet, the question I often hear is, "What can I eat for breakfast if you take my cereal, bread and oatmeal away?" I usually recommend trying a vegetable omelet with a side dish of cucumbers, tomatoes or asparagus—or any leftover vegetables from the night before. (Marinating the vegetables overnight in a sealed container in the refrigerator, after mixing them with rice vinegar or balsamic vinegar, will greatly improve their taste by the next morning.) Other options would be delicious green smoothies and soups. For more ideas and great recipes check out my book, *Your Best Investment: Secrets to a Healthy Body and Mind.*

Now, for the artificial sweeteners based on aspartame and sucralose, which are currently endorsed by the ADA for diabetics to use. Again, no surprise here, this is another controversial issue. The food industry profits greatly from the American sweet tooth, while the ADA bestows their blessing on aspartame, sucralose and other sweeteners.[1]

Aspartame

Aspartame is found in many foods and diet sodas. On a personal note, I was dependent for some time on diet sodas—drinking up to three cans a day. I later discovered that I was doing more harm than good. Aspartame has been linked to brain tumors, seizures, depression, headaches and neurotoxicity. Aspartame is composed of ten percent methanol, and methanol breaks down into deadly chemicals that the body has a hard time getting rid of—the most damaging of which are formaldehyde, formic acid and diketopiperazine (a known carcinogen).[2-7]

Now consider this. If you were to ingest some substance that contained 100 percent methanol (such as automobile anti-freeze), and didn't die (four ounces is fatal), you'd end up in the emergency room where they'd treat you for methanol poisoning with an ethanol intravenous drip. Now, think about all the ten percents of methanol you've consumed with aspartame—which does not have ethanol or pectin, so its methanol is converted into formaldehyde, formic acid and other harmful chemicals that tend to stay in your body. And, considering that aspartame is 200 times sweeter than sugar, it is much more appealing and addictive, thereby increasing its many adverse side effects! I strongly recommend that my patients avoid diet drinks and eliminate aspartame foods from their diet altogether.

Sucralose

But of even greater concern is sucralose, which is approximately 600 times sweeter than natural sugar, making it one of the main reasons many people are addicted to always wanting/eating something sweeter. Sucralose is a chlorocarbon, which is a chlorine-containing compound not found anywhere in nature. Sucralose is found in many different types of food including gum, mints and candy.

Amazingly, only two trials were completed and published before the FDA approved sucralose for human consumption. Unbelievably, those two published trials had a grand total of 36 total human subjects—and one trial only lasted four days!

Sucralose is approximately 15 percent absorbed after intake.[8] Its main danger is chlorine and the byproducts of chlorine. One of the byproducts of chlorine is dioxin, which is a 300,000 times more potent carcinogen than DDT (best-known as the potent pesticide used in the 1940s and 1950s, and now banned in the US).

For example, one of the largest industries using chlorine is the paper industry. They use it for bleaching paper to make it white. Since the long-term residual effects from chlorine are a public health concern, the American Public Health Association is trying to have the American paper industry use an environmentally friendly substitute. The byproducts of chlorine are dioxins and organochlorines, which are highly toxic and carcinogenic, especially to the environment.[9]

Unfortunately there is no long-term data or any trials on the safety or danger of sucralose. Eventually, when or if they are conducted, long-term studies for several years will be needed. I regrettably suspect that any future studies on sucralose will reveal long-term negative results.

"The proof is in the pudding."

In the first conversation I had with Dr. Lee regarding my newly diagnosed diabetes, I mentioned my concern for having to go down that well-travelled road toward insulin use. He reassured me that what he saw was a person that would not have to go down that road, and that my diabetes could be kept at bay with some changes in my lifestyle. At first it was a simple plan of watching what I ate and monitoring my blood sugars. Things seemed to go well, but I am a self confessed "foodie"—one that loves to cook and eat!

Over the last five months I've been following an approach suggested by Dr. Lee that, I will admit, for the first two weeks was tough; but I knew if I could do it one day at a time, then I could probably move on with it.

Well, "the proof is in the pudding," as they say. After the first six weeks my weight loss was 24 pounds. My other numbers were great as well. My A1C was now 5.5, my cholesterol ratio was 3.9 (never before had it been under 5) and to top it off my good cholesterol had gone to 44. That was the best ever recorded for me, and all these things mean better health for me. The praise from Dr. Lee came fast and with a smile.

Guidance and knowledge are very important tools in the battle we all face in order to reach and maintain better health. And it has been my good fortune to get my tools from Dr. Edwin Lee.

— Thomas Smekar

Blood Sugar

One amazing thing I've learned while working with my patients who have type 1 diabetes (their bodies produce neither insulin or the hormone called amylin), is that none of them can control their blood sugars after eating oatmeal or any other refined carbohydrates.

The device I use to monitor blood sugar is a continuous glucose monitor that tracks your blood sugar every five minutes via a tiny catheter inserted in your belly. The catheter—as small as a single hair from a horse—is inserted in the belly during an office visit (no surgery or knife needed). Then, once the continuous glucose monitor is working, you are provided with real-time data on your blood sugars. Diet has a tremendous influence on your blood sugars, and it is almost impossible to control the high spikes whenever consuming refined carbohydrates. Yet, thanks to continuous glucose monitoring and the real-time adjustment of diet needs that it provides, I consistently see type 2 diabetics enjoying a dramatic improvement in their blood sugars.

Back when I was working at the hospital, I remember helping many patients toward significant improvements in their blood sugars simply by adjusting their diets. One case that stands out in my memory is a 50-year-old male hospital patient who was on an insulin drip. He wasn't my patient, but I'd been asked to be a consultant on his case because, despite being on an insulin drip, his blood sugars were in the 300 range (whereas normal is less than 120 after eating, and less than 85 after fasting).

My timing couldn't have been better. As I walked into the room, I saw what this patient was about to eat. He was ready to take his first bite of this large sandwich on white bread. I also noticed the rest of his ADA approved diet for lunch: a can of diet soda, chips and canned fruit saturated in corn syrup. I immediately told him to stop and put the sandwich down. Needless to say, he wasn't happy that a doctor he'd never seen before had just interrupted his first anticipated bite of lunch. Then, I told him who I was and that I was going to help reverse his diabetes. He liked the sound of that.

I quickly learned that he was taking a kitchen sink of prescription medications for high blood pressure, cholesterol, anxiety, acid reflux and more. He agreed to change his diet right then and there, in the hospital. However, I then found out there were no fresh vegetables to be served in the hospital at all. So instead, I did the next best thing and put him on a vegetable soup diet, while making sure to alkalinize his drinking water with apple cider vinegar. In less than 12 hours he was able to get off his insulin drip! And the very next morning his blood sugar was under 130 without any insulin!

Unfortunately, some of the nurses thought I was starving the patient and so they gave him a grilled cheese sandwich that night and the next morning his blood sugar went above 250. At that point, I told him to please leave the hospital, read more about proper nutrition and then get back with me in one week. (To learn more about the dangers of having high insulin levels, be sure to read, *Your Best Investment: Secrets to a Healthy Body and Mind*.) Later, with that patient, I reintroduced whole grains into his diet while continuing with the high fiber.

The irony of the ADA advice on the treatment of diabetes is diet and exercise. It's the best advice but, unfortunately, it's failing since we are now one of the heaviest people in the world with an epidemic of diabetes in our youth.[10] The sad fact is that 80 percent of type 2 diabetes is preventable with proper diet, along with an increase in lifestyle activities.[11] It's failing for many reasons, but I believe one of the main reasons is that there is way too much advice on what to eat and how to eat—all of this conflicting advice becomes confusing, so people just give up.

"The Real Cost of Cheap Food"

Furthermore, I truly believe that in our society, the fast food industry and their high caloric poor nutritional foods are partly to blame. The cost of eating healthier is simply more expensive than eating foods from fast food restaurants that sell convenient and inexpensive quick foods of poor quality. In addition, how many commercials have you seen for eating more vegetables? Proof that the American media is the best in the world for selling anything. Education is the key to optimal health, but it's not a fair game when it comes to the food industry. Cheap foods that are high in calories and poor in nutritional value are, without a doubt, the number one reason for obesity in our country.

An article in Time Magazine on Aug 31, 2009 by Bryan Walsh, The Real Cost of Cheap Food,[12] revealed the dark side of the food industry and explored the true price of providing unlimited quantities of meat and grain—which comes at the expense of the environment, animals and us. Our farmlands are becoming depleted of nutrients, and our foods are becoming contaminated with pesticides, antibiotics and other chemicals. On top of that, the food industry requires more fossil fuels than any other industry, which is only escalating global warming.

In today's food industry, the animals are put in tight quarters and fattened up as fast as possible. For example, cattle are fed a corn-based diet and kept alive in prison-like conditions with the heavy use of antibiotics. Yet, despite the use of antibiotics, there are continued outbreaks of antibiotic resistant bacteria.

Also, the heavy use of fertilizers and chemicals that are used to increase crop production create a toxic runoff that contaminates waterways. In fact, because of those fertilizers and chemicals that are carried from streams to rivers to the Gulf of Mexico, there is a 6,000 square mile area in the Gulf where there is no oxygen and no sea life—but that 6,000 square mile figure was before the BP oil spill (the Deepwater Horizon oil spill) in the Gulf of Mexico. Around the world, there are approximately 400 similar areas—aquatic dead zones.

The best advice I can give anyone is to eat as healthy as possible. Eat organically, or eat from the land and sea. Do not eat from foods that are processed or that have chemicals or preservatives in them. If possible, try to grow your own herbs and vegetables. There is nothing better than when you eat from your own garden. Or, if you can't keep a garden, buy herbs and vegetables from your local farmers market or another reputable local source. When you can, buy meat that is grass-fed. If the meat is corn-fed, be sure that the feed is free of genetically modified organisms, pesticides, fertilizers, fungicides, herbicides, antibiotics and hormones.

To wash off any chemicals on your fruits and vegetables, and also to kill any bacteria, use pH water of 2.5 to kill the bacteria, followed by pH water of 11.5 to take away the fat-based toxins. Eating healthy does cost more, but in the long run it will pay off with better health. Remember let food be your medicine.

But that's getting harder to do, thanks to the growing controversy over genetically modified food. Unfortunately, approximately 60 percent or more of our corn, soybeans, cotton and canola are genetically modified. While the genetic materials that are inserted into plants or animals have desirable traits—like being resistant to insects, or an increase in beta-carotene production—the underlying concern is, what other genes are being genetically modified?

With genetically modified foods, safety is a major concern, and some organizations like Greenpeace argue there is not yet enough data on genetically modified foods to declare them safe to eat. A potential issue is whether or not genetically modified foods can trigger food allergies. Another possible side effect would be the spread of a gene from genetically modified plants to weeds—thereby creating super-weeds that are resistant to herbicides.

Obviously, there are more questions than answers when it comes to genetically modified foods. One of the best first steps would be to require the labeling of genetically modified foods; unfortunately, however, this is not required in the U.S. like it is in other parts of the world.

"I can't stop when I'm still winning races."

I am a 44-year-old professional triathlete. Since 1999, I've competed around the world. For the past several years, before seeing Dr. Lee, I was noticing that my energy and stamina were becoming very low. I was struggling with my training, and with my race performance. I felt burnt out, very emotional, and I had much self-doubt.

My triathlete friends told me to check out Dr. Lee, since he was a triathlete and would probably understood me better than any other doctor. And, because he had worked on many other professional athletes.

I have worked with Dr. Lee for several years now. Dr. Lee really achieved his goal with me, and that was better nutrition, and better absorption of nutrients. My energy and training are now back where I want them to be.

I keep telling Dr. Lee that this will be my last year to compete, and perhaps I will retire in another two or three years, but I can't stop when I'm still winning races, or placing in the top three.

If you want to improve your performance, I strongly recommend that you see Dr. Lee.

— Nina Kraft

Nutritional Guidelines

Simply stated, the most important part of nutrition is to eat as healthy as possible while avoiding any foods that are processed or chemically altered. The advice I give my patients every day for improving their energy is: eliminate the diet sodas, the artificial sweeteners and (for at least six weeks) the refined carbohydrates. The bad carbohydrates are rice, bread, pasta, potato, oatmeal, cereals, donuts, candy, grapes and oranges. Since no one is perfect, allow yourself a free day once every two weeks to indulge your food desires —within reason!

For the long run, I like a low glycemic diet for at least six weeks, followed by the reintroduction of whole grains—such as whole-wheat pasta, brown rice, sweet potatoes or whole wheat bread in small amounts. The key to improving your health and raising your energy level is to have more fiber and vegetables with each meal. I recommend two or three servings of vegetables per meal—including breakfast!

I used to eat cereal with a bagel in the morning, washed down with a glass of orange juice. But when I switched over, the amount of weight I lost, without even trying, and the energy that I had was amazing. Now, for breakfast, I love drinking a delicious green smoothie with protein powder or having lentil soup. Other suggestions for a vegetable breakfast include vegetable soup, vegetable omelet or hard-boiled eggs with two or three serving of vegetables. Again, for more ideas and great tasting recipes, please check out *Your Best Investment: Secrets to a Healthy Body and Mind*.

It is so crucial to avoid the refined carbohydrates—white bread, white pasta, white potatoes, white rice and foods with high fructose corn syrup (which all cause a spike in insulin)—to keep your blood sugars under control. The higher insulin levels can cause obesity, cancer, heart disease, depression and dementia.[13-15] In fact a low glycemic diet over six months will lower fasting insulin levels (a desired effect), lower blood pressure and lower cholesterol—as compared to patients on a high glycemic diet.[16] Carbohydrates are needed for energy production and also for your brain to work effectively—carbohydrates are the preferred source of fuel for the brain. However, it's all about the quality of carbohydrates, and for that you need to consume complex carbohydrates from vegetables, fruits with the skin (except oranges and grapes due to their high sugar content), beans, nuts and seeds—rather than from refined carbohydrates.

The carbohydrates from vegetables are an excellent source of fiber, minerals, vitamins and also phytonutrients. As a rule of thumb, I recommend consuming different color vegetables with each meal in order to maximize the power of the antioxidants from each unique vegetable. Also, consume four grams of omega-3 every day from a healthy source. These sources include walnuts, olive oil, flax seed, winter squash, fish, soy and beans to name a few. Omega-3 is a great source to decrease inflammation and to help with reducing your risk for cancer and heart disease.[17-20] As for protein, go with lean meats that are grass-fed, not grain-fed, and are raised free-range.

Vitamin Guidelines

A question that I get asked very frequently is, "What type of vitamins and minerals do I need to take?" So, I answer that question with, if you eat locally grown vegetables that are grown in nutrient rich soil, lean meats that are not grain-fed and are free from pesticides, herbicides, antibiotics and hormones, and are not genetically modified, and you are stress free and breath air that is not polluted and drink water that is totally chemical free, then you absolutely do not require any vitamins and minerals. For the rest of us, we require a high quality pharmacy graded multi vitamin and multi mineral.

There are several companies with tests to identify what nutrients in which you are deficient. The test I like to use when checking for nutritional deficiency also checks which amino acids, antioxidants and fatty acids that you may have a deficiency in. It also checks if you have oxidative damage, or DNA damage, which I consider a very important test to get done—as explained in Chapter 11.

The professional athletes I see in my office that complain of tiredness often have many different deficiencies. The athletes who are performing well usually have one or two deficiencies, while the ones not doing so well may have eight to ten deficiencies. Rarely do I ever find anyone who has no requirements for any vitamins or minerals.

"I finished that race faster than some of my 'no-cancer' friends."

As a triathlete with stage 4 cancer—and, undergoing chemotherapy and radiation treatment—my energy was wiped out. Fortunately, I was referred to Dr. Lee for help. After seeing Dr. Lee, my energy significantly improved, thanks to his weekly intravenous nutrition, combined with the supplements he prescribed. Then, after only two months of treatment, I not only was able to train, but I competed in the St. Croix International Triathlon.

In fact, I finished that race faster than some of my "no-cancer" friends. Thank you Dr. Lee!

— Maria D'Agostino

Unfortunately, a lot of physicians assume that we can get all of our nutrients from the foods we eat. Most physicians were not well versed in nutrition during their training. Even though I completed two fellowships after my residency training, I, like most physicians, really did not know much about nutrition. Because of this, I wish there were more classes in medical school to teach about the power of food in preventing many medical conditions.

The most common deficiencies I see in my patient are vitamin D, zinc, CoQ-10, vitamin C, and glutathione. I have seen many patients' energy levels improve from taking a great pharmacy grade multi-vitamin and multi-mineral, 2,000-10,000 units of vitamin D3 (depending on their blood levels), 20 mg of zinc, 100 mg of Coq-10, 2,000 mg of vitamin C, probiotic and 200 mg of N-acetylcysteine (the precursor of glutathione). I also recommend a high quality professional grade omega-3 for many of my patients. I prefer companies that are of professional grade, and have had medical studies performed on their products.

Vitamin D

Vitamin D is one of today's most popular vitamins because it has been shown to reduce cancer and heart disease.[21] Also, low vitamin D has been associated with an increase in autoimmune diseases like type 1 diabetes, systemic lupus erythematosus, arthritis and multiple sclerosis.[22] The role vitamin D plays in cancer is amazing. Vitamin D has even been found to induce death in cancer cells. A study by the National Cancer Institute found that a vitamin D level of 80 nmol/L or higher is associated with a 72 percent risk reduction.[23] In 2007, a double-blind, randomized, placebo-controlled study using 1,100 IU of vitamin D showed a reduction in all types of cancer by 60 percent within four years.[24]

The three sources of vitamin D are sunshine, dairy that is fortified with vitamin D and the ocean or plankton, which is the chief source of food for fish. Even practicing in Florida, I have diagnosed thousands of patients with vitamin D deficiency or insufficiency. The current debate in endocrinology is over the ideal level of vitamin D. Most endocrinologists are using about 1,000 IU a day of vitamin D, whereas I recommend an average dose of 5,000 IU a day (based on blood levels). Most laboratory data use a level of 20 to 100 ng/mL. I am recommending a level above 65 ng/mL in my patients to prevent cancer and to improve on energy. The most common side effect of too much vitamin D is nausea, vomiting or a kidney stone. Rarely, one can develop renal failure, which is why close monitoring is needed.

One incredible case of vitamin D deficiency that I saw was a world-class triathlete and mother of two. She was recommended to see a doctor by her coach, even after resting for a month. Her chief complaint was that she was exhausted and could barely run without feeling tired. Despite living in Florida and training outdoors, she had a severe vitamin D deficiency. She also had a progesterone deficiency, but after two weeks of treatment she was running faster than before. She is now a big believer in vitamin D and progesterone replacement.

To put this in perspective, consider what Hippocrates, the father of modern medicine, said more than two thousand years ago, "Let food be thy medicine." His sage advice is still true. It is critical to eat a high fiber, low glycemic diet with two or three servings of vegetables with each meal—and, if possible, try to eat your vegetables raw. Eating raw has many advantages, but it is not always easy. I would recommend starting off by steaming your vegetables, and then transitioning later to some raw vegetables. Also, avoid foods that come in a box since they are most likely processed and contain many preservatives and un- wanted chemicals.

Many of my patients have reversed their tiredness and regained their energy by including a digestive enzyme with each meal (in order to better absorb the nutrients they eat). In my practice, before I recom- mend spending more money on lab tests (nutritional evaluation test- ing), I recommend IV nutrition (more on this in Chapter 10) and deter- mine if it helps with low energy, or with whatever complaints they have. Most of my patients have significantly improved with IV nutrition; however, if someone is not responding, then I do offer a nutritional evaluation test.

As a rule of thumb, avoid diet sodas and artificial sweeteners, eat foods that come from the sea and land (not boxes), and you will significantly improve your health.

"We had the best time of our lives—with energy to spare!"

As a breast cancer survivor, I started coming to Dr. Lee six months after my last chemo. Dr. Lee did extensive research concerning cancer, and even presented me with a PowerPoint presentation. Now, after several urine tests, blood work and intravenous vitamins, my health is constantly improving.

My husband, Chuck, has been a patient of Dr. Lee's for the last ten years for his diabetes. Dr. Lee continues to treat Chuck for his diabetes and now, with the administration of growth hormone, Dr. Lee has been able to significantly decrease the amount of insulin Chuck uses. Plus, he now has a lot more energy and feels great.

A few months ago, we went to Las Vegas to celebrate our 29th wedding anniversary. Before we left we received our intravenous vitamins, and we had the best time of our lives—with energy to spare! Thanks Dr. Lee for caring about our health and helping us to feel great and age gracefully.

— Nancy and Chuck Young

Nutritional Supplements for Protecting DNA

As explained earlier in this chapter, telomere length has been correlated with the aging process.[25-26]

A recent study has shown that women taking a multivitamin had longer telomere lengths when compared to women not taking a multivitamin. It was also shown that the group of women who had a daily intake of vitamin C and Vitamin E had longer telomere lengths.[27]

A prospective study (with an average length of six years) of omega 3 was seeing if there was an association of telomere lengths in patients with heart disease. It was found that individuals with the lowest omega 3 levels had the fastest rate of telomere shortening over five years; whereas, the group of individuals with the highest omega 3 levels had the slowest rate of telomere shortening (the desired effect). Therefore, omega 3 intake is associated with prolonged survival in heart disease due to this positive telomere effect.[28]

In addition, another study has shown that higher Vitamin D levels are associated with longer telomere lengths.[29]

If I were you, I would be sure to at least take these three supplements: multivitamins, omega 3 and vitamin D.

"The importance of a balanced hormonal state, supplements and a proper diet."

For years I've recognized that there are inherent differences in how I perform versus my peers. Although I was always able to perform my operative procedures well throughout the day, in the evenings my energy levels were a lot lower. During the evenings, though, I felt as if I received a burst of energy after a power nap of ten to fifteen minutes.

I knew there was a problem, and so I mentioned it to my primary care physician who performed a battery of tests, including one adrenal test—a vanillylmandelic acid test. However, all my tests came back normal. There seemed to be no solution to my problem of feeling drained (which varied) and the fatigue (which was better with rest). I thought I had chronic fatigue syndrome. I tried some supplements, which I heard about through friends; however, the results were marginal at best.

Then I saw an advertisement in a local magazine about Dr. Lee and his practice called the Institute for Hormonal Balance. I didn't contact him right away, but when my symptoms got worse, I made the call and saw him. He was able to give me a brief synopsis of what he thought my problems were, which were soon confirmed with laboratory tests. I had adrenal insufficiency/ fatigue, confirmed by laboratory values to include low morning cortisol, afternoon cortisol higher than the morning level—but still overall low. That, without a doubt, explained the changes in how I felt.

He was able to provide me with natural supplements to affect the change. He also prescribed additional supplements, which were necessary—especially for my vitamin D level, which was very low, but is now within an acceptable range. Being at a certain age, my deficiencies were identified and the proper supplements were provided. Overall, I've noticed a dramatic difference in how I feel, and my outlook is much better because of my improved physical state.

I've made multiple recommendations for people to visit Dr. Lee because I do recognize the importance of a balanced hormonal state, supplements and a proper diet. Dr. Lee has made a world of difference.

— *Ivan G. Murray, M.D.*

CHAPTER 9 REVIEW

— If you want to lose weight and have more energy, then for six weeks you need to eliminate the "white sins"—avoid: bread, pasta, oatmeal, cereals, rice, potatoes, and dairy. Focus on having your largest meal in the morning, and your smallest meal in the evening. Increase your fiber intake by having two or three servings of vegetables per meal—including breakfast! Then, after six weeks, you may reintroduce whole grains into your diet.

— Avoid the artificial sweeteners aspartame and sucralose. These artificial sweeteners are addicting and are chemically altered to make you crave more carbohydrates.

— Avoid genetically modified foods, and try to eat foods that are organic. Eat as healthy as you can. By respecting your body and eating healthy, your body will enjoy huge benefits in the long run.

— If you want to know what nutrients in which you're deficient, have a nutritional evaluation test.

— A digestive enzyme, taken with meals, helps improve absorption of nutrients. I have seen many patients' energy levels improve from taking a great pharmacy grade multi-vitamin and multi-mineral, 2,000-10,000 units of vitamin D3 (depending on their blood levels), 20 mg of zinc, 100 mg of Coq-10, 2,000 mg of vitamin C, probiotic and 200 mg of N-acetylcysteine (the precursor of glutathione). I also recommend a high quality professional grade omega-3 for many of my patients.

— For more great tasting recipes that provide better nutrients, be sure to read *Your Best Investment: Secrets to a Healthy Body and Mind.*

10

Intravenous Nutrition

**"You can trace every sickness, every disease and
every aliment to a mineral deficiency."**
— Dr. Linus Pauling

The fastest and most effective way to improve on energy — and look
younger — is with intravenous (IV) infusions of vitamins, minerals,
amino acids and peptides. Although you could instead take all of those
vitamins and minerals by mouth (I have some patients who prefer to
take over 200 pills a day), the question is, how much is truly being
absorbed? Is it ten percent, fifty percent? The answer is, no one knows.

Yet, even though there is not yet a clinically available test to
determine how much of the vitamins and minerals you do absorb
orally, there is a test to see if you have DNA damage; which, in turn,
means that you have nutritional deficiency. From a simple blood or
urine sample, this test checks for 8-hydroxydeoxyguanosine (8-OHdG)
to determine the deficiency. In addition, for determining how healthy
you are, two other tests include the lipid peroxide test for cell
membrane damage, and the F2-isoprostanes test for oxidative stress.[1]

If there is DNA damage, the best way to repair such damage is with
intravenous vitamins, minerals and glutathione, which is needed by
the liver to help detoxify any toxins that are damaging your DNA.
Then, you can do a follow-up with another 8-hydroxydeoxyguanosine

(8-OHdG) test to determine your level of improvement. I have seen many patients improve after a series of IV nutritional therapies.

Glutathione, "Mother of All Antioxidants"

Most people—including some health care providers—have never heard of glutathione. (A low glutathione level is associated with cell death.) Glutathione is made of three amino acids: glutamate, glycine and cysteine.

Glutathione is considered to be the "mother of all antioxidants," and helps with the detoxification system in your liver. Glutathione is also considered to be neuroprotective against many neurodegenerative diseases such as multiple sclerosis, Alzheimer's and Parkinson's.[2-3]

The importance of glutathione was exemplified in a 2013 study on traffic police exposed to vehicular exhaust. The study showed that the traffic police had DNA damage (8-OHdG) associated with their years of service in traffic control. Specifically, a significant increase in DNA damage was indicated by the glutathione S-transferase gene defect— the gene that encodes the enzyme involved in the liver for detoxification, and which attaches glutathione to a free radical. Thus, in this study, vehicular exhaust over time (and other environmental toxins) resulted in an increase in oxidative stress (rusting in the body) and subsequent DNA damage.[4]

Because the mouth and stomach enzymes will destroy glutathione, it cannot be given orally. (Although, you may find glutathione pills being sold on the Internet.) As evidence of the inadequacy of oral glutathione, a recent study (a randomized, double-blind, placebo-controlled trial) was done on 40 healthy volunteers who were given 500 mg of oral glutathione daily for four weeks. There was no difference in oxidative stress markers, such as DNA damage (8-OHdG), and there was no improvement, or changes, in glutathione levels in the red blood cells.[5] Therefore, if you need glutathione, then you need intravenous glutathione.

A precursor of glutathione is N-acetylcysteine (NAC). NAC can be bought over the counter in a pill form for helping the liver detoxify better, and for helping increase glutathione levels. NAC is a derivative of the amino acid cysteine (one of the three amino acids that comprise glutathione); therefore, NAC can be used to boost glutathione levels. In fact, there are some promising NAC studies on depression, Alzheimer's and Parkinson's disease.[6-9]

Furthermore, in a 2012 study comparing eight elderly subjects to eight younger subjects, the elderly subjects—as expected—had lower glutathione levels, and higher markers of oxidative stress, when compared to the younger subjects. Then, when the elderly subjects received glycine and cysteine, their glutathione levels improved by an amazing 94 percent! In addition, their markers for oxidative stress improved dramatically. This study confirmed that nutritional support helps in decreasing oxidative stress of aging.[10]

Another study corroborating the use of nutritional support for the production of glutathione looked at twelve patients with poorly controlled diabetes. They all had low glutathione levels, and elevated markers of oxidative stress. The group received supplements of glycine and cysteine for 14 days; after which, it was shown that their glutathione levels improved, and their markers of oxidative stress also improved.[11]

Additionally, an older study (randomized single-blind design) used intravenous glutathione in ten diabetics who were not taking insulin. Before the treatment, it was noted that the diabetic group had insulin resistance and low glutathione levels when compared to healthy subjects. After the infusion of glutathione, their glutathione levels improved, and their blood glucose was lowered (desired effect).[12]

Another study (randomized, double-blind, placebo-controlled trial) looked at whether glutathione could protect against nerve damage (neuropathy) resulting from the chemotherapy of oxaliplatin. Fifty-two patients with advanced colorectal cancer were infused with glutathione (1500 mg) for 15 minutes before their infusion of oxaliplatin. The study proved that glutathione—an inexpensive antioxidant—had a significant reduction of nerve damage.[13]

Also, people with inflammatory bowel disease can benefit from IV nutrition, especially with glutathione. In a recent study, it was shown that patients with Crohn's disease have: oxidative stress in the intestine, high levels of the marker for inflammation (IL-6), and low levels of glutathione.[14]

And, in another study—this one being about NAC, the precursor of glutathione—it was shown in randomized, placebo-controlled research that taking NAC for four weeks improved in the treatment of ulcerative colitis, and it showed that the markers of inflammation were reduced.[15]

Not unexpectedly, glutathione's list of qualities is lengthy. Glutathione helps the liver detoxify better, and it helps with the immune system. As the "mother of all antioxidants," glutathione recycles all other antioxidants. Glutathione has also been shown to reduce inflammation, lower blood sugars in diabetics, reduce oxidative stress, protect DNA, protect the brain from oxidative stress and protect from the side effects of chemotherapy.[16-18]

Glutathione is also considered to have several positive effects for people with: chronic fatigue, heart disease, autoimmune disease, liver disease, Alzheimer's, Parkinson's and many other conditions.[19-20]

I can only say that I consider glutathione to be simply amazing.

"I haven't felt this good since my 20s!"

When I first visited Dr. Lee, I was 39 years old and my symptoms were: extreme fatigue, depression, insomnia, anxiety and severe memory issues. I had gone from being a top salesperson for a decade in biotech sales, to losing my job and having to sell my home.

I was sleeping 18-19 hours a day. I couldn't work. I didn't even have the energy to take a daily shower. I cried and had anxiety attacks almost daily.

Before meeting Dr. Lee, I had gone to four different doctors who ran dozens of tests and told me I was "fine." I had given up hope. During my first visit with Dr. Lee, he sat with me for more than an hour. He took a detailed history of my health—beginning when I was 15 years old. He listened carefully and promised that we would figure it out and that I would feel better. I felt hopeful for the first time in years. He started me on bioidentical hormones twice daily, had me give up all foods and drinks with "diet" chemicals in them, and had me start getting an IV twice a week.

Now, I am exercising for the first time in years. Most days I don't even take a nap. My depression and anxiety have subsided. I even occasionally win at the game of Memory against my seven-year-old nephew! I haven't felt this good since my 20s!

I have made it my mission to tell as many people as possible about Dr. Lee. My mom and several of my friends now see him. They have gone to him for an assortment of reasons, and they have all had similar success stories. Dr. Lee and his team gave me my life back, and for that, I will never be able to fully express my gratitude.

— Stephanie Jones

Dr. Linus Pauling

One of the most famous American scientists that ever has lived was Dr. Linus Pauling. A two-time Nobel Laureate, Dr. Pauling famously said, "You can trace every sickness, every disease and every aliment to a mineral deficiency." Unfortunately, after his death, the medical establishment branded Dr. Pauling a quack (thankfully, for only a few years) because of his belief that high doses of vitamin C can treat many diseases. (Supplementation of vitamin C is necessary since humans cannot manufacture vitamin C.)

The controversy over vitamin C began in 1976 when Dr. Pauling went on record about using high doses of vitamin C in the treatment of cancer.[21] Later, in 1979, there was a Mayo Clinic study to confirm whether or not vitamin C had any effect on patients with advanced cancer.

Unfortunately, that study was not done with <u>intravenous</u> vitamin C, as Dr. Pauling had done. Furthermore, the patients were given only 10 grams of oral vitamin C, which was far less than Dr. Pauling's recommended dosage.

Nonetheless, and regardless of its inconsistencies and shortcomings, the study was published in the New England Journal of Medicine. Because of that article, vitamin C was, for a few years, mistakenly branded as useless.[22]

Now, almost 20 years after Dr. Pauling's death, there is an abundance of scientific data confirming the health benefits of vitamin C—ranging from treating the common cold, to adjuvant treatment of cancer, to improvement of the immune system. There was even a recent study that showed vitamin C deficiency was present in patients with advanced cancer. (As mentioned earlier, humans cannot manufacture vitamin C.) Furthermore, it was noted in the study that the patients' lower vitamin C levels were associated with their shorter survival rates.[23]

What's Your Current Level of Vitamin C?

Knowing now, as Dr. Pauling knew, that an intravenous infusion achieves a much higher level than an oral dosage, how would you prefer to increase your level of vitamin C?

I personally know that intravenous vitamin C works on the common cold. When I feel like I could be catching a cold, I give myself some IV vitamin C. I usually feel much better in less than 24 hours. Combining zinc with <u>IV vitamin C</u> also helps, as shown in a 2012 article on the benefits of vitamin C with zinc in treating a cold.[24]

Another 2012 article showed that high doses of intravenous vitamin C (up to 50 grams) helped reduce markers of inflammation (CRP, IL-2, TNF and others) in a wide range of cancer patients.[25]

In a phase one clinical trial with IV antioxidants (that included IV vitamin C), the IV antioxidants were proven to help patients with chronic hepatitis C. This was an interesting study in that it was seeing whether or not the antioxidants could help reduce the inflammation of the liver caused by the virus. In hepatitis C, the virus causes inflammation of the liver cells, which leads to oxidative stress, and then death of the liver cells. The IV antioxidants (vitamin C, glutathione and vitamin B-complex) showed on histology (under the microscope) that the liver cells improved and that the viral load of hepatitis C was reduced. No major side effects were noted.[26]

In a study on diabetes, it was shown that intravenous vitamin C provided clinical improvements in diabetic patients. It was a small study, which is why I would love to see a larger study to determine vitamin C's effect on diabetes—since diabetes is a state of chronic inflammation.[27]

Also, there have been many reported studies and cases of intravenous vitamin C helping in the treatment of cancer.[28-29]

For example, in a phase one clinical trial on patients with metastatic pancreatic cancer, it was shown that intravenous vitamin C with chemotherapy was safe, and there were no adverse side effects.[30]

There is even a theory that vitamin C kills certain cancer cells—due to vitamin C helping in the production of hydrogen peroxide, which can cause cancer cell death.[31]

Another study has shown that intravenous vitamin C helped improve the quality of life for breast cancer patients undergoing chemotherapy and radiation therapy.[32]

To conclude this section on IV vitamin C, I'd like to share a story. After one of my patients received IV vitamin C, he felt better that afternoon, and quickly overcame his flu-like symptoms. He later told his wife, who is a news anchor and, before I knew it, she had me on camera, discussing why intravenous vitamin C is decidedly better than taking vitamin C by mouth, or drinking a lot of orange juice.

While it does help, of course, to take vitamin C orally or drink orange juice, the key point is that intravenous vitamin C is estimated to be "50 to 70" times stronger than vitamin C taken by mouth. In addition, intravenous vitamin C is 100 percent in the veins, immediately ready to be utilized by your cells.

One contraindication to receiving intravenous vitamin C is if you have a glucose 6 phosphate dehydrogenase (G6PD) deficiency. A G6PD deficiency is a genetic disorder that can be detected by a simple blood test. People with a G6PD enzyme deficiency can develop a reaction where their red blood cells burst (hemolytic anemia) if they take a certain medication, or a high dose of intravenous vitamin C. At normal levels, G6PD keeps the red blood cells functioning properly; however, a G6PD deficiency reduces the production of glutathione in the red blood cells. Any excessive oxidative stress on the red blood cells with a G6PD deficiency, combined with low glutathione levels in the red blood cells, can cause the red blood cells to burst. Before receiving a high dose of intravenous vitamin C, you should have this test done.[33-34]

"IV treatments are really making the difference."

Our primary care doctor referred me to Dr. Lee after unsuccessfully trying four different doctors for pituitary, thyroid and adrenal insufficiency. I am 71, and was having many miserable symptoms including: weakness, tiredness, poor mental focus, no endurance, nausea, and I was not having mental clarity. Always feeling exhausted and woozy, with poor orientation and balance, was debilitating and depressing.

Now, the IV treatments are really making the difference. I have more energy, endurance, and normal functioning—for which I am so thankful.

After today's IV treatment, I felt so great that I walked rapidly for 35 minutes, rode my bike for over 7 miles, did some work, and I still feel great while I'm writing this at 8:39 p.m. Normally, just the exercise would have reduced my energy by 50 percent, but I am not tired and am still raring to go. It is the best I have felt in many years. Just today, others have said I have more life and my skin and color look better. Not bad for 71.

You have really given me my life back. Thank you so much Dr. Lee!

— Bill Baumner

Magnesium

Magnesium is an essential mineral that is involved with more than 300 biochemical reactions in the body—including, significantly, the production of energy (ATP).

Included among magnesium's many positive effects on the body are: helping the liver detox better, helping with body temperature regulation, improving muscle contraction, helping insulin to work more efficiently, aiding in protein synthesis and assisting in the absorption of calcium.

IV magnesium is used extensively in emergency rooms and in critical care units across the United States.

I remember my days in critical care medicine, when I used a lot of IV magnesium to help treat cardiac arrhythmias. IV magnesium is also used to treat asthmatic attacks and preeclampsia,[35-37] and has been shown to rapidly alleviate various types of headaches.[38]

I have seen the benefits of IV magnesium help with headaches, and with high blood pressure (magnesium helps in vasodilation of the blood vessels). In fact, in a recent emergency room study, it was shown that IV magnesium is an effective blood pressure agent.[39]

Phosphatidylcholine (PC)

Although there are many more nutrients I could discuss, the last one I want to mention here is phosphatidylcholine (PC). PC is a fat, or lipid, in the cell membranes of your body's 100 trillion cells. PC is also found in your proteins. PC is the main source of a neurotransmitter of acetylcholine. Alzheimer's is the main cause of dementia, and one of the causes of Alzheimer's is the loss of acetylcholine.

PC is necessary for the production of surfactant for your lungs and gastrointestinal tract. Before the discovery of surfactant, many prematurely born infants died due to the absence of lung development. A well-known case was the second son of President Kennedy. The infant, Patrick Kennedy, died only two days after he was born 5½ weeks premature in 1963. Fortunately, these days, there is surfactant for premature infants.

PC is the major lipid found on the mucosal layer (the layer which interacts with the digestion of food) in the intestinal tract. In a study (a randomized, double-blind, placebo-controlled trial) on patients with active ulcerative colitis, it was shown that PC therapy provided improvement in their quality of life and—most significantly—a 90 percent rate of clinical remission.[40]

PC has also been shown to help patients with chronic liver disease;[41] although, this was a small study, and I would now like to see more research in this area.

In another study on Alzheimer's, almost 900 men and women, over the course of nine years, were studied for the risk factor for developing Alzheimer's disease. This extensive research determined that those found to have a higher level of PC, also benefitted with a 47 percent less risk for developing dementia.[42] I believe that an interesting study for the future would be on the effects of intravenous PC in the early stages of Alzheimer's.

Although there are not many clinical trials to prove the benefits of the use of PC (beside that of surfactant), it is significant to note that PC, as one of the key ingredients in your cell walls, is one of the most important structures for keeping your DNA healthy in each and every one of your body's 100 trillion cells.

While your younger body can produce PC from the fish, eggs, meat, milk or wheat germ, your older body produces less. Given that we are learning more about DNA, and the cell walls that protect it, I have confidence that future studies will further confirm the benefits of PC.

I strongly believe that, as we age, we become more nutritionally deficient. This, oftentimes preventable, process of nutritional deficiency can result in damage to your DNA—damage that can lead to premature aging, chronic disease, cancer and early death.[43]

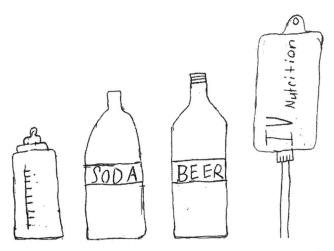

It has been said that, as we age, we graduate from one of these to the next; although, not everyone does so at the same pace!

Artwork by Connor Lee (nine years old) and Nathan Lee (eight years old).

As a side note, three of the most important additional ways for improving on oxidative stress (DNA damage) are to: optimize and balance your hormones, find and fix the source of any chronic inflammation you are experiencing, and do a liver detox to help your body get rid of fat-soluble toxins. (To learn more on detoxification, see Chapter 11.)

Additional Benefits of IV Nutrition

The many benefits of IV nutrition programs are often described by patients as life-changing. Each of the IV nutrition programs at my office are individually tailored for each patient. Additionally, the programs can be specifically modified for: boosting energy, improving your immune system, lowering blood pressure, improving circulation, improving brain fog, treating a cold, slowing degenerative vision loss, and reducing the symptoms of multiple sclerosis.

Although most people feel much better with IV nutritional therapy, there may occasionally be a patient who will only feel a minor improvement, not feel anything at all, or have a minor reaction. Overall, the majority of my patients enjoy a remarkable improvement when they receive IV nutrition.

IV nutrition works as an infusion of vitamins, minerals, amino acids and other nutrients into the blood stream. A small catheter is inserted into the vein, and is connected by a plastic tube to a bag filled with the appropriate nutrients. This is the most effective and powerful way to deliver nutrients to your body and brain.

Sometimes, the absorption of nutrients from your stomach can be very poor—and no matter how much you eat or drink, you may not be getting more than 10 percent of that total intake into your blood system. Plus, as you get older, the absorption of those nutrients from what you consume will become even worse.

As I said at the beginning of Chapter 1, the phrase, "You are what you eat," would be much more accurate as, "You are what you absorb." You can take over 100 different vitamins or supplements by mouth, but if you are not absorbing them, it is a waste of time and money.

However, when you get IV nutrients, you are getting 100 percent of the nutrients into your blood system. From there, the nutrients are delivered to all the cells in your body.

"Feeling like I did many years ago."

Before Dr. Lee, I was not very healthy. I was on multiple medications for blood pressure and I was feeling unmotivated, tired all the time and fatigued. Dr. Lee had me do a liver cleanse, and then an IV program and testosterone.

Now, at 54, I am off all but one of my medications, my blood pressure is way down, and I'm feeling like I did many years ago. My wife and kids have told me they can tell I am so much more active, happy and that I like myself again. Thank you Dr. Lee. I look forward to my continuing journey with you.

— Joe Floyd

IV Therapy Guidelines

IV nutrition therapy presents a powerful way to help your body at a cellular level to become more efficient, and to repair itself from the effects of the toxic environment in which you live. Therapies that help repair the damages you encounter are called regenerative medicine. IV nutrition therapy is the cornerstone for regenerative medicine.

It is important to find a physician knowledgeable in intravenous vitamins and minerals replacement. The physician needs to know the total osmolarity of the fluids that are given, they need to avoid any significant hypertonic or hypotonic fluids, and they need to be ready in case there is a rare side effect of an anaphylactic shock.

While this is rare, it can happen. For example, if a person who is allergic to corn is receiving vitamin C that is corn derived, they can have an acute reaction.

Regarding the improvement of energy, most people feel better after several intravenous cocktails. Although, for some, it may take until the eighth or tenth treatment before they feel significantly better.

"It was not until I started getting IVs that my energy returned."

In 2009, I was forced to retire early because I no longer had the energy to do my job. One doctor had even diagnosed me with chronic fatigue syndrome. I pretty much slept, ate and stayed on the sofa all day, moving around enough to care for only my most basic needs. I had tried many, many approaches over the years, but finally I felt my body had given out and all I was good for at age 59 was to watch television and mourn my lost life.

Shortly after retiring, I first visited Dr. Lee. He took a thorough history, read my previous reports and really listened to me. I remember dragging myself into his office and thinking, "Can he really help me?" It took a little while to see results. Dr. Lee balanced my hormone levels, suggested supplements to take and tested me for food sensitivities, but it was not until I started getting IVs that my energy returned. Specifically, he gave me detox IVs for my liver that included antioxidants and vitamins.

Within a few weeks, I was a new person. Instead of riding carts through stores, I was easily walking through them. Driving an hour each way to and from Dr. Lee's office no longer wore me out. I started getting involved in volunteer work that fulfilled me, and even took a Spanish course so I could help at a free clinic. Now, at 63, I am able to do one-hour Pilates sessions, and instead of watching game shows on television, I am auditioning to be a Jeopardy contestant. Thank you, Dr. Lee!

— Kathleen Riley

Recommended IV Therapies

IV therapies at the Institute for Hormonal Balance may range all the way from ten minutes, up to four hours. For the most part, IV therapies in my office last from thirty minutes to one hour. Initial treatment courses usually consist of ten to twenty IV therapy sessions, with monthly follow-up treatments. Some of the IV therapies I recommend are:

Detox (30 minutes)—Great way for your liver to detoxify and get rid of toxins. Key ingredients include glutathione, calcium, B12, magnesium and B-complex.

Wellness Modified (60 minutes)—Exceptional way to improve on energy. Excellent for pre-operation and post-operation. Helps with hair loss, and for people with poor absorption of nutrients. Key ingredients include 15 grams of vitamin C, B-vitamins and minerals.

Minerals (45 minutes)—Vital for people with heart problems, diabetes, autoimmune diseases, heavy metal toxicity, and memory issues. Key ingredients include higher dose of magnesium, Calcium, trace minerals and B5.

Vitamin C (2 hours/50 grams of vitamin C)—Perfect for treating the common cold or a virus. Great antioxidant, plus it helps with increasing energy and reducing inflammation.

Glutathione Push (5 minutes)—As the "mother of all antioxidants," glutathione is the most important ingredient for the liver to detoxify. Great for many conditions ranging from IBS, chronic fatigue, diabetes, autoimmune disease, heart disease and liver disease.

Phosphatidylcholine Push (5 minutes)—Phosphatidylcholine is the most important nutrient for your cell walls. This quick IV is ideal for neurodegenerative disorders like MS, Parkinson's, high cholesterol, skin disorders and memory disorder.

"I compare my experience with IV therapy to a
wilting flower given water to come back to life!"

I am 34 years old and had seen many different doctors before Dr. Lee. When I came upon his practice, I was looking for help with fatigue, brain fog and other female hormonal issues. He found that I had hypothyroidism and a progesterone deficiency. Soon, with bioidentical hormone replacement therapy, I was back to my old self.

I also began IV therapy for high dose Vitamin C, B-vitamins and minerals. I compare my experience with IV therapy to a wilting flower given water to come back to life! After five treatments, I could think more clearly, I had more energy and clearer skin, and my days were much more productive. Also, I now have greater endurance and fewer muscle aches during and after exercise.

Dr. Lee gets to know all aspects of his patients' life for holistic health... mind, body and soul. He spends much more than the typical five minutes with you, unlike other doctors. He truly listens and wants you to feel your best, which means he doesn't just look at normal or abnormal ranges on a blood test, but weighs that along with your symptoms and how you feel. It's great to see a doctor whose top priority is to make you feel, think and look your best, and whose approach is for prevention to keep you healthy and strong, while avoiding disease in the years to come. Dr. Lee is a doctor with a sharp mind and a big heart!

— *Angela Luster*

CHAPTER 10 REVIEW

— Intravenous nutrition is the most effective way to improve upon your energy, and look younger, since your cells need nutrients to work better.

— Accelerated aging is due to chronic inflammation and oxidative stress that can cause cell wall damage and DNA damage.

— Glutathione has been shown to reduce inflammation, lower blood sugars in diabetics, reduce oxidative stress, protect DNA, protect the brain from oxidative stress and protect against side effects from chemotherapy.

— Vitamin C is an amazing antioxidant, and has been shown to help with overcoming the common cold, reduce inflammation, help against certain cancers and hepatitis.

— Before getting an intravenous vitamin C, you should be checked to see if you have a glucose 6 phosphate dehydrogenase (G6PD) deficiency.

— Phosphatidylcholine (PC) is essential for cell wall health.

11

DETOXIFICATION

The liver is the most under-appreciated
organ in our bodies.

An important part of reversing tiredness is optimizing your detoxification system. We live in a toxic world thanks to all the processed foods, chemical exposures, pesticides, herbicides, smoke exposures, artificial chemicals and preservatives to which we're constantly being exposed. Exercise helps in sweating out some of those toxins, and daily bowel movements are extremely important as well.

Likewise, the liver, kidney and colon are important organs in eliminating those toxins, as well as the chemicals not needed by your body. In fact, I believe that overall, the liver is the most under-appreciated organ in our bodies. The liver takes fat-soluble toxins and chemicals and modifies them so either the kidneys or colon may then excrete them. If all the toxins were water-soluble, then your urine could carry them out of your body. However, most environmental toxins are fat-soluble and must be cleared through your liver.

In 1947, R.T. Williams described the liver's detoxification process in two steps. The first step is phase I, which uses oxygen to modify the toxin. Then, in phase II, the liver adds another chemical (conjugation) so that it becomes water-soluble. Then it can be excreted through the kidneys or through the bile, which later goes through the colon or stool.[1]

During phase I, the liver primarily uses the enzymes called cytochrome P450. Most of your pharmaceutical medications are metabolized through phase I. Oxygen is primarily used in the phase I detoxification pathway. This process makes a free radical (makes a more toxic molecule than the original toxin). If this free radical is not further metabolized by phase II's detoxification pathways in the liver, then this can increase the risk for cancer, Parkinson's and other diseases.[2-4]

By the way, the most important antioxidant for neutralizing these free radicals is glutathione. Again, phase II detoxification involves conjugation, which adds a compound that binds to the toxin—such as glutathione, methyl, cysteine or sulfur.

Constipation

Those that are constipated and have bowel movements less than once or twice a day are not able to clear toxins out of their bodies. The metabolic waste and toxins in the stool accumulate in the stool and can also ferment and produce other toxic byproducts.

These byproducts, toxins or steroid hormones can then reenter the bloodstream and overload the body, thus causing tiredness, illness and even cancer. An increase in your fiber or vegetable intake can help with constipation. The high fiber has been shown to lower estrogen levels, thereby lowering the risk of breast cancer.[5-6]

Detoxification and Cancer

An example of the importance of your body's ability to properly detoxify is the danger of developing breast cancer. Your liver is a very important place where estrogen is metabolized or detoxified. The estrogen can then either go along the good pathway or the bad pathway, depending on the health of your liver.

The breakdown of estrogen is then sent to your bowel to be excreted. When stool remains in the bowel for a long time, as in constipation, the estrogen is reabsorbed. The excessive estrogen then increases the stimulation of breast tissue, which increases your risk for breast cancer.

According to the Journal of the National Cancer Institute, it has been shown that high levels of 16 alpha hydroxylated estrogens (bad estrogen that is excreted from the liver) increase the risk of breast cancer.[7] In a recent 2009 study, it was shown that high levels of the 16 alpha hydroxylated estrogens (bad estrogen) increase the risk of breast cancer.[8]

Furthermore, another study showed that lower levels of the 16 alpha hydroxylated estrogen (bad estrogen) will lower the risk of breast cancer.[9] A simple test to screen for breast cancer (although it is not the only cause for breast cancer) is a 24-hour urine test to look at the ratio of the good estrogen and bad estrogen (2-hydroxyestrone/16alpha-hydroxyestrone ratio). This test also looks at how the liver is metabolizing or detoxifying the estrogen. If you have undesirable levels of the 16 hydroxylated estrogen or 16alpha-hydroxyestrone (bad estrogen), then there are natural ways to convert your bad estrogen to good estrogen.

Another concern about this toxic world we live in is that girls are reaching puberty earlier than they used to. The average age used to be around eleven to thirteen years, and now it can be as young as eight or nine. There are many theories about the cause of the higher exposure to estrogen. Some of the theories range from the plastics in water bottles, to cosmetics, to contaminated water supplies (for example, birth control pills flushed down the toilet), to the hormones being used in the food industry.[10]

Some of the chemicals are polybrominated biphenyls (PBBs, chemical flame-retardants), dioxins, phthalates and bisphenol A (commonly known as BPA), which was originally developed as a synthetic hormone, but is now used in all polycarbonate plastics and the linings of food and beverage cans.[11]

Aside from the fact that these girls are losing part of their childhood due to advanced puberty, this is of major concern because early puberty is a risk factor for developing breast cancer. These endocrine disrupting chemicals, which mimic hormones, are also linked to obesity and diabetes.[12]

Smoking

As most people realize, smoking is one of the worst habits to have. Smoking not only increases the risk of lung cancer, heart disease, asthma, stroke and lung disease, but it will rob your energy by accelerating your aging process.

According to the American Cancer Society, smoking causes one in five deaths.[13] Smoking is the single largest preventable cause of disease and premature death. Just by smoking, the body is burdened with the undue process of handling nicotine, carbon monoxide, formaldehyde, arsenic and lead—to name a few. One of the reasons that smoking can cause many problems is that it triggers inflammation, and the markers of inflammation are then elevated—like CRP, TNF and IL-6.[14]

Nuclear factor kappa beta (bad blood marker) is also increased by smoking, which is the centerpiece for inflammation.[15] Nuclear factor kappa beta is a protein or a small molecule that controls the transcription of DNA. In other words, nuclear factor kappa beta is considered a first responder to any harmful cellular stimuli, or to inflammation, and when activated it can call for back up.

If the nuclear factor kappa beta is over activated, then this can turn on more severe inflammation (like throwing gasoline on a fire), which can cause cancer, arthritis, inflammatory bowel disease or autoimmune disease. The good news is that if one quits smoking then the signs of inflammation will be lowered.[16] However, it is impossible to reverse tiredness if one still smokes.

Open That Spigot!

Analogically speaking, your body is like a barrel with a spigot on the bottom of that barrel. Your body, or the barrel, can only handle so many toxins from processed foods, chemical exposure, pesticides, herbicides, smoke exposure, artificial chemicals and preservatives.

The spigot represents your ability to get rid of those toxins, and if you take in more than you can get rid of, then your body is due to fail. The barrel will overflow with toxins and these toxins can then be stored in your fat, or in your brain. These accumulated toxins can cause chronic inflammation and damage your DNA, which can lead to chronic disease, tiredness, developmental disorders, neurotoxicity and cancer.

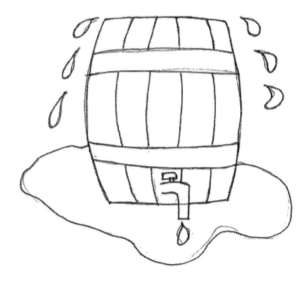

In this concept of an overworked liver, the barrel represents your liver. If the barrel's spigot is not maximally opened, or if more toxins (alcohol, smoke, pesticides, herbicides, preservatives, etc.) are put into the barrel than the barrel can handle, it will overflow toxins and free radicals into your body. This overflow of free radicals will damage the most important structure in your body, and that is your DNA.

Artwork by Connor Lee (nine years old).

The best way to open up your spigot as much as possible is to improve the different routes of elimination available to your body — like your kidneys, skin (sweating), liver and daily bowel movements. In addition, hormonal balance, exercise, laughter, vitamins, proper nutrition, minerals, enzymes, amino acids and antioxidants will help.

The ultimate therapy is intravenous therapy, which can guarantee absorption and bring the essential vitamins, minerals (needed for phase I liver detox) and especially glutathione (needed for phase II liver detox). In the process of removing toxins out of your body, this will result in lowering inflammation and subsequently help your cells produce more energy. This approach will definitively help to reverse your tiredness, while helping you to achieve optimal health.

"Treatments had failed everywhere — including the Mayo Clinic."

I walked into Dr. Lee's office lacking enough energy to get through my day as an active physical therapist and mother of two small children. Several auto-immune disorders and hormonal imbalances had begun to dominate my life after treatments had failed everywhere — including the Mayo Clinic.

Dr. Lee's careful evaluation started me on a plan that finally has my energy level improving. In conjunction with medication changes, he started me on IV nutrition therapy and IV detox that has changed my life! For the first time in years I can get through a work day, and I've even been able to start exercising again. I only wish I had found Dr. Lee sooner!

— Katherine Strauss Brandt

Oxidative Stress

An excellent way to measure if you are healthy and have a great detoxification system is to measure for your oxidative stress. The test I like to use for measuring oxidative stress is the 8-hydroxy-2'-

deoxyguanosine (8-OHdG), which is a critical biomarker of oxidative stress, carcinogenesis and DNA damage.[17]

As you may recall, your liver has two pathways called phase I and phase II. Oxygen is primarily used in the phase I detoxification pathway. This process either makes a free radical, or it makes a more toxic molecule than the original toxin. If this free radical is not further metabolized by the phase II detoxification pathways in the liver, then this can increase the risk for cancer, Parkinson's and other diseases.[18-19]

Other sources of oxidative stress are exposure to cigarette smoke, irradiation, environmental pollutants and infections. In addition, oxidative stress is linked to cardiovascular disease since oxidation of the bad cholesterol (LDL) in the blood vessels forms plaque and atherosclerosis.[20] High levels of the 8-OHdG have been shown to correlate with the severity of Parkinson's disease.[21] In another study, there was evidence that increased levels of 8-OHdG were found in brain sections from patients with neurodegenerative diseases like Alzheimer's disease, Huntington disease, frontotemporal dementia (FTD) and Pick's disease—as compared to control subjects.[22]

Environmental Toxins

A study in Jordan has shown that exposure to large environmental toxins—like the exposure received by chemical factory workers, paint workers, gasoline station workers and smokers—showed that an elevated 8-OHdG is a predictor for sudden coronary death.[23]

Another point to emphasize about the dangers of oxidative stress is that an elevated 8-OHdG in diabetics is a marker for complications.[24] Whether the 8-OHdG (a sign of oxidative stress or a marker for DNA damage) will be accepted in conventional medicine is still up for debate, since the topic of detoxification is far from being accepted.

Again, it all goes back to the analogy of the barrel and spigot. If your spigot cannot drain fast enough, your barrel overflows with toxins, and you'll be in trouble because the ensuing chronic inflammation and excessive oxidative stress can only lead to many problems—including chronic disease, cancer and DNA damage.

By maximizing the opening of your spigot (with hormonal balance, proper nutrition, exercise, laughter, vitamins, minerals, antioxidants and IV therapy), you can reduce oxidative stress and improve on the detoxification system of your liver. Once you've "opened your spigot," all you have to do is repeat an 8-OHdG test to have quantifiable results of your improvement.

Sadly, even with quantifiable results, such as the 8-OHdG test, many conventional doctors—who, unfortunately, did not receive training in medical school on detoxification—do not know how important it is to tell you to detoxify.

The ultimate irony is that while conventional doctors know smoking leads to cancer, and they will tell you to remove cigarettes from your life, they also know that toxins lead to cancer, yet they resist the evidence for telling you to detoxify.

This is something that needs to change.

"I have achieved a total body balance
I never dreamed possible!"

With the help of IV detox treatments, bioidentical hormone therapy, and vitamin and mineral supplements, I have finally achieved a total body balance I never dreamed possible!

And, thanks to my success with the Institute for Hormonal Balance, my son, who is currently a sophomore in college, now receives IV detox treatments as well. We had tried many methods to keep him from constantly becoming sick with food allergies, etc.; but now, under Dr. Lee's care, our son has not had any illnesses, and he credits Dr. Lee with his success—in and out of the classroom. I can finally see the light at the end of the tunnel!

— Mary Lee Hollis

CHAPTER 11 REVIEW

— We live in a toxic global environment, thanks to all the processed foods, chemicals, pollution, pesticides, herbicides, smoke, artificial chemicals and preservatives to which we're constantly being exposed.

— Your liver is crucial in converting the toxins your body receives — converting them from fat-based, into water-based, so that you can excrete them from your body, instead of allowing them to reside in your fatty tissue.

— If your liver is weak, then toxins and free radicals are generated more often than eliminated, which can lead to DNA damage.

— The liver uses a 2-step process known as phase I and II. Phase I adds oxygen to the toxin but generates a free radical. Phase II neutralizes the free radical by adding a sulfur, methyl, glutathione, glucuronic acid, acetyl or amino acid; thereby neutralizing the free radical and converting the fat-based toxin into a water-based toxin, ready for eliminating.

— The key to feeling good and having a healthy life is having a strong liver that works, or detoxifies, well.

— There are special tests to determine if your liver has an adequate phase I and phase II. Most of the patients I check usually have an extremely weak phase II.

— Hormonal balance, exercise, laughter, vitamins, proper nutrition, minerals, enzymes, amino acids and antioxidants will help your liver detoxify better.

— The ultimate detoxification therapy is delivered intravenously and contains minerals, vitamins, glutathione and other proteins that guarantee absorption and help the liver to better detoxify.

12

EXERCISE

**"We do not stop exercising because we grow old —
we grow old because we stop exercising."
— Dr. Kenneth Cooper, The Cooper Institute**

Most doctors today will agree that exercise has positive effects, and exercise is recommended by the American Heart Association, American Diabetes Association and others. The benefits of exercise do reduce chronic inflammation, and exercise does lower the markers of inflammation — such as C-reactive protein (CRP) and TNF.[1]

One of my biggest pleasures in life is simply going outside and exercising. I enjoy the outdoors and especially the fresh air. I often wonder why I love to push myself to see how far and how fast my body can take me. I do know that one of the reasons I enjoy to exercise is that I find the body is the most amazing piece of machinery there is, and that we all have the ability to enjoy its benefits.

However, I realize that not everyone is like me. I don't expect any of my patients to participate in triathlons or to run marathons. But I do expect that if you want to reverse tiredness, then you have to invest in your health by spending at least 30 minutes a day in a physical activity that you enjoy.

> *"His understanding of the athlete's mentality*
> *is a huge plus for those of us who count*
> *on our active lifestyles to keep us sane."*

I am a 49-year-old female distance runner and I have competed in many races, including several marathons over the past few years. I love to run and it is a very important part of my lifestyle.

This past winter, after a busy racing season, I competed in the Gasparilla Half Marathon with a terrible case of plantar fasciitis. Bumping into my friend (and sometimes running buddy) Dr. Ed Lee at the finish line, he noted how badly I was limping. We talked a minute and he gave me his direct number with instructions to call him on Monday.

Dr. Lee told me about a treatment delivery system called Hybresis™. He arranged for my appointment right away with a physical therapist. I received treatment twice a week for a little over a month and was able to continue running throughout the process. By the end of the treatment, my pain was completely gone and I have not been troubled since.

I owe many thanks to Dr. Lee. His understanding of the athlete's mentality is a huge plus for those of us who count on our active lifestyles to keep us sane. We do not want to be taken "off the road" for any reason! I will continue to seek out Dr. Lee for injury advice or improvements on my performance.

— Holley Simoneau

The Dangers of Overtraining

The old saying that, "Too much of any one thing is not healthy," is so true, especially when it comes to overexercising. Even I have experienced some adrenal fatigue, some oxidative damage and many other injuries from too much exercise.

Overexercising is one of the worst things you can do to cause premature aging. Examples of overexercising include: burning over 4,000 calories per day, training for more than two hours per day, or doing more than one marathon or one Ironman in a year.

By overtraining (overexercising), you will increase oxidative stress and develop many free radicals that can: damage your DNA, weaken your immune system, or burn out your adrenal glands. Overexercising is an addiction and I was an addict for many years; however, since I became a dad, I am learning to enjoy a different chapter of my life.

For some of the people I see in my practice, I don't have to worry about them overexercising. I would be happy if they did any type of activity at all. I truly believe that where there's a will, there's a way.

No More Excuses!

Many times I hear people say they just don't have the time, or they admit to just being lazy—sometimes they go as far as to admit, "I'm just a lazy bastard!" I really think the key in exercising is the mindset that exercise can be fun. It should not be a chore, but something that you look forward to. For me, I can't wait until each weekend morning because that's when I bicycle, swim a mile in a lake, or run before the sun comes up. Sometimes it's a special treat if I can do all three in one morning! Exercise is one of my favorite activities, and I become somewhat depressed when I can't exercise regularly.

For those using the excuse that they travel a lot or they just don't have time to exercise, I often think of a particular surgeon that invited me on a morning run. I often run at 5:30 a.m. but when he invited me for a 4:30 a.m. run, I thought he was crazy. But this surgeon loves to run and usually works over 14 hours a day, or more, yet he still finds time in his busy schedule to run almost daily. In life, if you want to achieve a goal, then you will have to work at it. I really believe if you want it then you will find a way to get it. It's all about how bad or how deeply you want something.

Because I have traveled a lot, I do know the stresses that come with traveling, but I always find a way to exercise. The easiest way is to bring your running shoes and explore the new world around you, even if you sometimes get lost—though I do enjoy the challenge in trying to find my way back.

Another way to exercise while traveling is with a swim cord that you attach to a stationary item by the pool, like a ladder, and then attach the swim cord's Velcro® straps around your ankles. With this, you can swim in place by converting a small pool into a treadmill for swimming. On one of my trips, I swam a mile every day on a cruise ship in a little heart-shaped pool. The little pool made it impossible to swim laps, but the swim cord allowed me to swim in place, giving me a great 20-minute workout.

Another idea is to join a gym with multiple sites where you can go, or just pay the daily fee to work out. I've been in many different gyms in many different countries by just paying a nominal fee.

"With energy to spare!"

At the age of 39 I was diagnosed with chronic fatigue syndrome. I had seen many different doctors and my daily activities were virtually impossible to perform without experiencing complete exhaustion. But, since working with Dr. Lee, I can now participate in pump classes and in yoga.

In fact, I can now do anything I desire—with energy to spare! I have my life back and feel like I am in my twenties again.

— Lori Levine

Exercising to Reverse Tiredness

Exercise is key to reversing tiredness, but it also has other benefits. Exercise promotes better sleep by helping you fall asleep faster. It also improves your sex life by increasing the blood flow to your sex organs. Not to mention that regular exercise promotes more energy and helps you to look better.

One of the best benefits of regular physical activity is weight loss/ control. Many patients that I have seen have lost an extra 15 to 20 pounds by living a more active lifestyle. Another benefit of exercise that I enjoy is blowing off steam. If I am stressed out, my wife usually tells to me go for a run. Then, when I come back, I'm calmer and my mind feels more relaxed thanks to the endorphins that are triggered into release by exercise. I also find that while exercising, I can reflect back on the day or take time to think about some ideas. Exercise is key to avoiding chronic disease like heart disease, diabetes, osteoporosis, colon and breast cancer and high blood pressure. There are many other benefits of exercise—like improving your mental focus, improving on your good cholesterol level and lowering triglycerides, increasing your strength and stamina, improving your digestion and improving your circulation.

Startup Guidelines

Of course, it is important that you get a blessing from your physician if you are out of shape and are considering starting an exercise program. It is also important to take a stress test with an electrocardiogram and a recovery electrocardiogram to make sure you do not have a cardiac problem. Also, find out what your 85 percent maximum heart rate is, and never exceed it when you are first working out. Wearing a heart monitor helps you keep tabs on your heart rate when doing any cardiac activity.

A simple and commonsense piece of medical advice is to quit smoking in order to obtain the full benefits of exercising. A friend of mine who smokes wanted to get in shape, so I started coming to his house in the morning for a light jog three days a week. After a month he started to go a little further and a little faster. However, at the end of each run, he was always gasping for air. I simply told him you don't have to suffer like that... all you have to do is quit smoking.

A simple, startup exercise plan is to walk for 20 minutes a day, and then try to walk for 30 minutes a day, five days a week. Later, when you're more comfortable with the walking, try some interval workouts by walking fast for two minutes, then walking normally for two minutes, then repeat the fast walk and normal walk cycle several times. As my patients progress, I'll have them increase their intensity and endurance while reminding them to have fun and enjoy the process of it all.

My advice when exercising is to focus on five key areas: cardio with interval workouts, strength training, balance exercises, flexibility exercises and core exercises. For example, when a new patient says they've been doing an hour on the treadmill but they can't lose any weight, I switch them to high intensity anaerobic interval workouts of 20 to 30 minutes—which then result in weight loss. Furthermore, a Vo2 Max test is needed to be done to calculate what heart rate needs to be achieved to lose weight. (See Vo2 Max testing later in this chapter.)

Since I have been injured multiple times and have spent many sessions in physical therapy, I have learned the hard way the importance in being flexible. All of my sport related injuries were from being as tight as a thick rubber band, which is why it is crucial to learn to stretch—and a great way to stretch and become flexible is by doing yoga. I love yoga. It has helped me tremendously in becoming more flexible, and it helps me relax. I'm still working on my flexibility, but already I'm more flexible than I was in high school.

To prevent injuries, it is important to warm up and stretch before any exercise—and afterwards, while your muscles are still warm. For me, my problem area has been tight hamstrings (the back of my legs), but by stretching every day I have become more flexible. While this does require an extra investment of time, it will reward you tremendously in the long run.

"I have always been very close to my wife, which makes it hard to believe how much better we get along now that we both feel great!"

Thank you, Dr. Lee! I'm feeling the best I've felt in years, and loving life! At my wife's recommendation, and after witnessing the miracles you did for her hormonal imbalances, I made an appointment. Honestly, I didn't think I had any problems. I thought because I exercised and ran several marathons, that was pretty much all I needed to do. However, after reviewing my blood work, you made me realize I had quite a few issues that needed attention.

After applying your recommendations for changing some of my exercising and eating habits, doing a fast, adding supplements and testosterone therapy, I've lost ten pounds and feel healthier than I did in my thirties! The high intensity anaerobic running workouts that Dr. Lee recommend (basically, it's running fewer miles at a faster pace) really helped me lose the extra weight.

I've been married for 37 years, and I have always been very close to my wife, which makes it hard to believe how much better we get along now that we both feel great!

— Blaine Vermeulen

Running

For those who enjoy walking, jogging or running, I highly recommend going to a specialty running store that can professionally fit you in a running shoe or a walking shoe that fits your particular stride. It is important to be fitted, and to find a shoe that does not cause injuries like blisters, loss of toenails or plantar fasciitis.

The real key, however, is proper running form. It's like learning a proper golf swing will help lower your golf score, or developing an efficient swimming stroke will help you swim faster. Two books on proper running form that I recommend reading are *Pose Method® of Running* and *Born to Run: A Hidden Tribe, Superathletes, and the Greatest Race the World Has Never Seen.*

Another recommendation is to change your shoes after 350 to 400 miles, or when the bottom of the shoe is degrading. Also, run more on the front of your foot—avoiding heel to toe.

You can wear old shoes to run, but then it's like driving a car with worn out tires. Sometimes I find that when patients hate to jog, it's because they get injured a lot, and then we learn the injuries were due to their worn-out running shoes.

Vo2 Max Testing

One of the reasons many people struggle with their weight—despite regular exercise—is they may not be exercising in a way that brings their heart above their own unique anaerobic threshold. They may be at the gym for 2 hours a day, and sweating profusely, but not losing weight because their exercising heart rate is simply not fast enough to burn fat.

Your anaerobic threshold is defined as the point when your body has switched from its aerobic (oxygen plus) state, to its anaerobic (oxygen debt) state, which is when you will begin to successfully burn fat.

At my office, we determine your anaerobic threshold on the same machine used at the National Olympic Training Center—and at Duke University, University of Florida and John Hopkins. The machine and its equipment are known as the Vo2 Max test. In a very sophisticated way, it tests your cardiovascular fitness. Interestingly, some of my weight lifter patients (only the ones who neglect working out their cardiovascular system) have done poorly on this test.

The Vo2 Max test will last about 10 to 12 minutes. The only uncomfortable thing you may experience is having to breath into a tube while your nose is pinched. This is needed to measure your expired gases. At first, the bike ride will be easy; however, it will become more difficult every several seconds, and you will eventually reach your anaerobic threshold—which is when you begin to generate certain levels of lactic acid and carbon dioxide. Once you reach that anaerobic threshold, the Vo2 Max test is nearly done. From that point, you will simply continue for as long as you can. You may only last another minute or less—and that is okay—but you do need to give it your 100 percent best effort.

In explaining how the V02 Max test determines your anaerobic threshold, I typically use this money analogy: Crossing your anaerobic threshold is like when you go from having money, to going into debt. In the beginning of a Vo2 Max test, you start off with money (glucose and glycogen). During the Vo2 Max test, you accumulate expenses (the building up of carbon dioxide and lactic acid). Your body wants to pay those bills (rid itself of that excessive carbon dioxide and lactic acid) by using up all your cash (glucose). Once you use up all your cash (glucose) then you start dipping into your cash reserve (glycogen). Eventually, you will use of all your cash reserve (glycogen) and you will tap into a new source of energy (fat), since there is no more glucose or glycogen. This is your anaerobic threshold—where your body starts burning fat for energy. Every person has their own unique anaerobic threshold. There is no cookie cutter formula to determine it.

Then, armed with the results of your Vo2 Max test, I will create a customized workout for you that will be 20 to 25 minutes long, three times a week. The rest of the week you can do other activities, but just be sure to do your customized Vo2 Max workout three times a week, and no more than six times a week.

This customized workout is what Olympic and professional athletes use, and it will help you burn fat and lose weight.

Strength Training

Strength training is as important as doing cardio exercises and stretching. So that you can train properly—and prevent injuries— strength training should be done with a personal trainer if you are new to it. Two of the strength training exercises I would recommend are pull ups and squats. I would also recommend doing core, or abdominal, workouts to help build up a strong core.

Working out with weights is a great way to build up your muscles by causing micro-tears in your muscles that your body then repairs by building up stronger muscles. Working with weights also helps build up stronger bones, improves on muscle endurance, improves on posture, improves on the immune system and makes you less prone to low back injuries. But, most importantly, remember that...

...in order to build up your muscles properly, you first have to be hormonally balanced and be receiving the proper nutrients.

Notice how we keep coming back to that? How so very much depends on the basic requirements of hormones and nutrition?

"Dr. Lee is my hero,
but I still want to crush him in the next race!"

I'm a 52-year-old mother of 12-year-old twins, who is passionate about competing in triathlons. I've been active all my adult life, but have become increasingly involved in the sport in the last eight years.

I've steadily improved, have raced all over the US, and have been able to compete in three International Triathlon Union Long Distance World Championships in Europe and three Ironman 70.3 World Championships. I've been a USA Triathlon All American, which is a ranking in the top 10 percent of all triathletes, of all distances, for the past 7 years.

When I was starting in triathlon, I developed a fun rivalry with Dr Lee. He is a much better swimmer and would always try to help me. I returned the favor by trying to track him down on the run. I've never succeeded, but I've gotten close!

In the fall of 2007, I was a little tired and my race results were suddenly much slower. For example, my run, which is my strength, in the Ironman 70.3 World Championship was seven minutes slower than the previous year! I had similar results in both a ten mile race and a half marathon road race.

My coach, Jeff Cuddeback, suggested that I see a doctor and have some blood work done. Dr. Lee ran several tests and discovered that I was deficient in vitamin D. I simply started taking vitamin D, and after a few weeks felt like myself again. Before the vitamin D, when I was tired, I couldn't break a seven minute mile. Three weeks after starting vitamin D, I ran a six minute mile — in the middle of a run!

I turned 50 in April of 2008 and decided to celebrate by competing in Ironman Lake Placid. The Ironman consists of a 2.4 mile swim, a 112 mile bike ride and a 26.2 mile run. It turned out to be quite a celebration as I had the race of my life! In the pouring rain, I had a good swim and bike, and was in tenth place. I then ran past 491 other racers, seven of whom were in my age group. I placed third and earned a slot to the Ironman World Championships in Hawaii—my very first Ironman! I also ran fast enough after biking and swimming to qualify for the Boston Marathon. I competed in Hawaii ten weeks after my first Ironman, and again had a good run! I managed to pass ten people in my age group and ended up 14th, again qualifying for Boston.

I am so relieved and excited. I was worried that my speed was gone forever. The surprising thing is that I am continuing to get faster at age 52—in my ninth year in the sport! Dr. Lee is my hero, but I still want to crush him in the next race!

— Julie Sands

Start Today!

We were all given a gift of an incredible machine, our body. If you treat it well, then it will treat you well. You have to keep your body in shape and respect it. Your job is to do daily exercises or regular physical activity, and to enjoy it. It's important to stay flexible, do some cardio with your interval workouts and to do some weight training.

So, start today—not tomorrow—and enjoy the process of it. You will reverse tiredness with regular physical activity, and you may also lose weight on the road to improving your energy. One day perhaps, we may meet while hiking up a mountain, kayaking, swimming, running, cycling or snowboarding.

CHAPTER 12 REVIEW

— It is important to obtain your physician's approval before beginning an exercise program. It is also important to take a stress test with an electrocardiogram and a recovery electrocardiogram to make sure you do not have a cardiac problem.

— Stretch before, and especially after, working out to keep your body loose. When you stretch, it is important not to bounce, but to go slightly into discomfort, and never into pain. Yoga is a great place to learn how to become more flexible.

— Strength training is important for building muscle, strengthening bones and burning fat. Remember to work on the back part of the body, which is often neglected, by doing squats and deadlifts. If you are not familiar with an exercise, then I recommend consulting a personal trainer.

— Interval workouts are great for burning calories, and for improving your heart and lungs.

— We were all given a gift of an incredible machine, the human body. If you treat it well, then it will treat you well. You have to keep your body in shape and respect it. Your job is to do daily exercises, or regular physical activity, and to enjoy it.

— Vo2 Max testing is an excellent test to determine what heart rate you need to achieve in order to begin burning fat. Most people, despite regular exercise, do not get their heart rate fast enough to burn fat.

13

SLEEP

**"When I woke up this morning,
my girlfriend asked, 'Did you sleep good?'
I said, 'No, I made a few mistakes.'"**
— Steven Wright

Even if you are reducing chronic inflammation, addressing adrenal fatigue and following my other directives to help reverse tiredness, if you are not getting seven to eight hours of sleep every night, your body is missing out on one of its most natural and needed essentials.

Not surprisingly, many of my patients are also struggling with poor sleep quality—often complaining that they can't turn off their minds when going to bed, have trouble falling asleep, wake up several times during the night or simply wake up exhausted.

"One of his first questions was, how was I sleeping?"

I am a 56-year-old woman who started seeing Dr. Lee almost two years ago when I wanted to talk about bioidentical hormone replacement for my hot flashes. After intently listening to me explain my issues, one of his first questions was, how was I sleeping?

Since I never was a good sleeper, I never gave much thought to my sleeping patterns. I just thought, as we got older we slept less. I'd always had a hard time getting to sleep, and would often wake up during the night, not able turn off my mind.

He explained to me how important sleep is because that is the optimal time for your hormones to reproduce, and without that happening, I will never get my hormones balanced. With some lifestyle changes and Dr. Lee's expertise, I now go to sleep, am able to sleep through the night and wake up refreshed.

My husband also sees Dr. Lee, as he was not sleeping due to stress from his job. I am happy to report that he is now sleeping through the night. We are both enjoying our life more since we're sleeping better, thanks to Dr. Lee.

— Nancy Clairmont

Melatonin

While there are several medical conditions contributing to insomnia, one of the most common is a low melatonin level. Melatonin is a hormone produced in an area of the brain called the pineal gland. However, the pineal gland's production of melatonin begins a continuous decline after the age of five. Consequently, there are even children with sleep problems! Fortunately, there are medical studies showing that melatonin therapy works in children and adults with chronic insomnia, and that it is safe to use.[1-3]

One can check for melatonin levels with a saliva melatonin level test or through the urinary excretion of melatonin, but I prefer to empirically use sublingual or under the tongue melatonin to see if you can benefit from it. In my experience, I've found that sublingual melatonin has helped many patients.

Progesterone

Another condition that can help with insomnia is the use of progesterone. Progesterone deficiency is a common condition that is often overlooked in the conventional medical community because it is typically only thought of as the hormone that's important for pregnancy. However, progesterone is one of my favorite hormones that helps many of my patients to sleep better and also to achieve inner peace.

I often prescribe progesterone under the tongue (sublingually) so that it can dissolve directly into the bloodstream and bind to the GABA receptors (the chief inhibitory neurotransmitters in your central nervous center) to help patients sleep better and reduce anxiety.[4] As mentioned earlier in the chapter on progesterone, I even have my male patients on sublingual progesterone—two of the reasons are for better sleep and anxiety reduction.

"I believed that I was a heart attack in motion."

I am a 43-year-old podiatrist from Virginia, and after talking with my sister-in-law, who recently saw Dr. Lee, I decided to invest in my health. I started to see Dr. Lee in 2009. I was in private practice, a new mother, a wife and homemaker with extreme fatigue. Feeling burned out, combined with the effects of perimenopause, had begun to take its toll. I couldn't sleep, suffered from extreme fatigue, hot flashes, mood swings and weight gain—and these were just a few of my problems!

I believed that I was a heart attack in motion. I know Dr. Lee's focused attention and his willingness to think outside the "medical box" has given me quality of life back. He has diagnosed me with severe adrenal fatigue and also with progesterone deficiency. I now sleep like a baby with sublingual progesterone. I also have more energy than ever, even outlasting my five-year-old son during an all day adventure at Disney World. I feel like I have recaptured my health. I thank Dr. Lee for his guidance, and I now know that I will live a longer, happier and healthier life.

— Dr. Renee P. Mazzei

Sleep Apnea

Another serious medical condition relative to insomnia is sleep apnea.   Sleep apnea can present itself with excessive daytime sleepiness, loud snoring, headaches, excessive urination during the nighttime, memory loss, low sex drive and, of course, tiredness. The most common sleep apnea is called obstructive sleep apnea, and it occurs when an obstruction of the upper airway is present, resulting in a very dangerous period (or a pause) of not snoring or breathing. We can live without water and food for a few days, but we cannot go very long without oxygen.

The most common risk factor for obstructive sleep apnea is obesity. To diagnosis sleep apnea, a sleep study is conducted to monitor how many pauses of breathing you experience during a typical night of sleep. Once identified, the treatment of obstructive sleep apnea may vary from wearing a special shirt so that you do not sleep on your back, surgery to open up any anatomical areas of obstruction, or wearing a continuous positive airway pressure (CPAP) or bilevel positive airway pressure (BiPAP) while sleeping. After having been tested for sleep apnea, I was diagnosed with mild obstructive sleep apnea. Now, thanks to wearing a BiPAP machine while sleeping, I've noted significant improvement in my energy.

Depression

Another cause of insomnia is depression. Depression is a symptom of a root problem or problems. Although the medication class of selective serotonin reuptake inhibitors (SSRIs) has helped many people with depression and insomnia, it really is just a band-aid over the problem. The SSRI raises the serotonin levels in the brain that helps with depression and anxiety disorders. I have used SSRI in some of my patients to help with acute depression and with insomnia. But, the bigger question is, why do depressed people have low serotonin levels?

In conventional medicine, if you have depression, you are placed on the path of taking antidepressants and may be committed to take them for a very long time. In conventional medicine, it is unthinkable to say that depression may be linked to the gut. Depression has also been associated with the leaky gut syndrome through the leakage of gram-negative bacteria. This "turns on" the immune system, which triggers inflammation, which is then followed by an elevation of IL-6 and TNF (bad blood markers). Significantly, tryptophan is used up during this period of chronic inflammation, which leads to a lower level of serotonin, which is the root cause of depression.[5-6] Proper sleep can also reduce the inflammatory markers like CRP and IL-6.[7-8] Is it not truly amazing that something like a problem in your gut can cause depression? Consequently, if you don't fix the gut then you won't reverse the depression.

Other Factors

My friends in neurology who are board certified in sleep medicine recommend that you remove the television from your bedroom. This may be painful for many people out there, but it is crucial to obtain seven to eight hours of undisturbed sleep every night. I also recommend that you try to relax one or two hours before bedtime, and to turn off the phone and television at that time.

Another problem that I see is with patients who have a pet that requires constant attention throughout the night, robbing them of their undisturbed sleep. It's a tough decision, but if you want to take care of others, then you need to take care of yourself first.

For those patients watching the late, late talk shows or for those that go to bed around 2 a.m., they need to slowly re-adjust their biological clocks. I often recommend that those patients try to fall asleep 30 minutes earlier, and over time, gradually working toward obtaining seven to eight hours of undisturbed sleep every night.

Sleep deprivation may even be a cancer risk according to some medical studies. What is worrisome is that people working the night shifts or doing night shifts for long periods of time may increase the risk of developing cancer.[9]

In conclusion, it is so important not to burn the midnight oil frequently and to get the proper amount of sleep. One may require progesterone, 5-hydroxytryptophan (5-HTP) to increase the serotonin levels and/or the use of melatonin. Another topic to investigate is leaky gut or delayed food sensitivity to certain foods that can be linked to insomnia. These conditions are linked to inflammation in the gut and with an increase of "bad" bacteria in the gut that uses up tryptophan and thereby lowering your serotonin and melatonin levels, which causes insomnia.[10-11]

By the way, the best sleep that I have ever experienced as an adult was after a strenuous hike of 37 miles over two days in the Grand Canyon. Upon reaching the canyon floor, I fell asleep around 8 p.m. right next to the Colorado River. It felt like Mother Nature rocked me to sleep that night, and I was a new person the next day.

"He looks at the whole picture, rather than just treating the symptoms."

I started seeing Dr. Lee eight months ago for chronic insomnia. After a thorough analysis, Dr. Lee put me on various vitamins and hormone supplements, and for the first time in several years I am sleeping through the night. My energy level is better, my moods are more stable and most of all I am finally getting a good night's sleep.

I truly appreciate and value Dr. Lee's approach to health care in that he looks at the whole picture, rather than just treating the symptoms. Thank you Dr. Lee for everything.

— Vashon Sarkisian

CHAPTER 13 REVIEW

— A good night's sleep is one of the best things you can do for your body and mind. Improving sleep is the first step in improving on energy.

— Proper sleep can restore adrenal fatigue and help with improving the active growth hormone, IGF-1.

— Progesterone taken under the tongue can help with insomnia. Progesterone binds to the GABA receptors of the brain to help with calming the brain and to help with sleep. Also, the use of melatonin under the tongue can help with insomnia.

— Ask your sleep partner if you stop breathing while sleeping or if you snore a lot. If so, or if you don't know, then you may need to have a formal sleep study to evaluate for sleep apnea.

— Another source of insomnia is the deficiency of amino acid tryptophan, which is used up by gram-negative bacteria from a leaky gut syndrome, which leads to a lower level of serotonin and thus, a lower level of melatonin. (Melatonin is the hormone involved in sleep.) In this case, if you fix the gut, then you fix the brain as well as the insomnia.

— It is very important not to burn the midnight oil frequently, and to get the proper amount of undisturbed sleep. Most people need seven to eight hours of undisturbed sleep.

14

LAUGHTER

**"You can fake an orgasm
but you can't fake laughter."
— Bob Dylan**

Appropriately enough, I'd like to open this chapter with three of the funnier stories from my fifteen years in private practice.

— *One of my patients was having trouble remembering the name of his recent medical procedure. Then, a little later, meaning to say, "biopsy," he said he remembered and that his procedure had been an "autopsy."*

— *This story helps illustrate just how devoted my patients are to their total wellness. While one of my patients was filling her car's tank with gas, she was approached by two young thugs who demanded her car keys. She calmly gave them the keys and told them the car was all theirs. But as soon as they jumped in, they jumped right back out and ran away... when her German Shepherd stood up from the back seat. Then, some other customers at the gas station who'd seen what happened volunteered to call the police to report it, but my patient said, "I don't have time for paperwork—I'll be late for yoga!"*

— *Once, when a patient asked if she had a leaky gut, I embarrassingly mis-spoke when I replied, "Yes, you have a leaky butt."*

Just saying that laughter is beneficial to your health is nothing new. It was written in Proverbs 17:22, "A merry heart doeth good like a medicine; but a broken spirit drieth the bones." Yet, while there's no doubt that laughter feels good, is there any real scientific basis behind that feeling; and, more importantly, what can we do about it?"

Proof of Laughter's Benefits

In a paper presented to an American Physiological Society session at Experimental Biology in 2006, Dr. Lee S. Berk of Loma Linda University reported that not only is there real science and neurophysiology in laughter, but just the anticipation of the "mirthful laughter" involved in watching a funny movie has some very surprising and significant neuroendocrine hormonal effects.[1] In other words, just knowing you're probably going to be laughing, your body begins "salivating" like Pavlov's dog at the anticipated benefits!

According to Dr. Berk, "The blood drawn from experimental subjects just before they watched the video had 27 percent more beta-endorphins and 87 percent more human growth hormone, compared to blood from the control group, which didn't anticipate the watching of a humorous video. Between blood pulls, the control group stayed in a waiting room and could choose from a wide variety of magazines." Dr. Berk then stated that the strong difference between the two groups in terms of human growth hormone (HGH) and beta-endorphin blood levels was maintained from just prior to the beginning of video watching, throughout the hour of viewing and continued long afterwards.

"We believe the results suggest that the anticipation of a humor/laughter event initiates changes in neuroendocrine response prior to the onset of the event itself," Dr. Berk explained. He further noted, "From our prior studies, this modulation appears to be concomitant with mood state changes. And taken together, these would appear to carry important, positive implications for wellness, disease-prevention and most certainly stress-reduction."

Earlier experiments showed that viewing a favorite funny video can offset symptoms of chronic stress, which can suppress various components of the immune responses, particularly those related to anti-viral and anti-tumor defenses. In addition, there appears to be a rebalancing of the Th1/Th2 (different types of T helper cells) immune response, which suggestively could lead to reduction of autoimmune issues.

"Laughter diminishes the secretion of cortisol and epinephrine, while enhancing immune reactivity. In addition, mirthful laughter boosts secretion of growth hormone, an enhancer of these same key immune responses. The physiological effects of a single one-hour session viewing a humorous video has appeared to last up to 12 to 24 hours in some individuals," Dr. Berk noted, "while other studies of daily 30-minute exposure produces profound and long-lasting changes in these measures."

Future research in this area with more subjects "needs to elaborate these findings in psychoneuroimmunology understanding and the mechanism linkage modulation between anticipatory positive behaviors and neuroendocrine and immune responses," Dr. Berk concluded, "It may sound corny but we in the health care medical sciences need to 'get serious about happiness' and the lifestyle that produces it—relative to mind, body and spirit and its biotranslation."

The "Biology of Hope"

By now, you may have noticed the lack of any patient testimonials in this chapter, which is probably indicative of the quality of my jokes that I tell my patients. Nevertheless, I do try to interject humor into my time with my patients. As I've learned over the years, I do believe that happiness and laughter are the "biology of hope," and, much like my belief that hormones should never be synthetic, laughter should be real too. Or, as Bob Dylan said best, "You can fake an orgasm but you can't fake laughter."

Which reminds me of something I mentioned earlier in the testosterone chapter, and I would like to once again reference, but with a little more information. It was a case where I had the privilege of evaluating a male physician who was experiencing tiredness, loss of libido and weight gain. During his work-up he noted that he used to have a lot of energy, but over the past several years his energy had been slowly decreasing. He also noted that he had gained some weight, or belly fat, which was hard for him to lose. Testing indicated that his testosterone was very low and he was experiencing some early bone loss. Rather than just using testosterone, I had him do a special test to see whether his pituitary gland (in the middle of the brain) was working well.

Within four days of this test he knew that testosterone was what he was missing. Then, with therapy to increase his testosterone level, he soon started reversing his tiredness while regaining his libido, his weight control and... his sense of humor. Later, he told me that the best thing of all was regaining his sense of humor.

That story always reminds me that Dr. Seuss was exactly right when he said, "Nonsense wakes up the brain cells. And it helps develop a sense of humor, which is awfully important in this day and age."

So, I'll keep trying to get it right with my doctor-patient jokes; however, I've already got it right when it comes to knowing how truly vital it is to just be happy and count your blessings daily.

CHAPTER 14 REVIEW

— Anticipating, and then watching, a funny movie has been proven to increase human growth hormone (HGH) and beta-endorphin levels—which are positive implications for wellness, disease-prevention and stress-reduction.

— I do believe that happiness and laughter are the "biology of hope," and, much like my belief that hormones should never be synthetic, laughter should be real too. Or, as Bob Dylan said best, "You can fake an orgasm but you can't fake laughter."

— Dr. Seuss was exactly right when he said, "Nonsense wakes up the brain cells. And it helps develop a sense of humor, which is awfully important in this day and age."

15

ENERGY PRODUCTION

**"The higher your energy level,
the more efficient your body.
The more efficient your body, the better you feel
and the more you will use your talent
to produce outstanding results."**

— Tony Robbins

While there is no magic pill for reversing tiredness, I often focus on hormonal balance, gut health, liver detox, better sleep and better nutrition. All of these topics have been covered in detail in the previous chapters, but if you can get all five of these optimized, then you will receive significant improvement in your energy production.

Sometimes, all it takes is a simple ten day liver cleanse, one or two hormones, some simple nutritional supplements or an IV therapy, and by the next follow-up appointment, your energy level may improve from a three (out of ten), up to an eight in less than a month. Although I have worked on some patients who may take a little longer, each time they do feel better.

Regarding hormones and energy, the main topics are: sex hormones (estrogen, progesterone and testosterone in women, testosterone in men); adrenal fatigue; low thyroid (or an imbalance of Free T3 with Reverse T3); high insulin levels (see *Your Best Investment: Secrets to a*

Healthy Body and Mind to learn more about the dangers of insulin resistance); and low growth hormone. I usually start by addressing the sex hormones (women start with progesterone and possibly estrogen, then testosterone later), then evaluating for adrenal fatigue. I do a complete blood and saliva test for adrenal fatigue, and for other hormonal issues.

The best way to diagnosis adrenal fatigue is to do a four-point cortisol test (morning, lunch, dinner and bedtime). This allows you to see the different patterns of cortisol levels—and the treatment depends on the cortisol pattern.

One of the best treatments for adrenal fatigue is to sleep more and have a better quality of sleep. I see so many patients that struggle with insomnia, or have been "burning the midnight oil" for too long. There are many natural supplements that will help you sleep better, and I often use a mixture of them. Progesterone under the tongue is also wonderful to help people sleep better and I sometimes use this for men, but in much lower doses than I use for women. Sometimes, I refer patients for a sleep study to see if they have sleep apnea.

Along with better sleep for adrenal fatigue, I use supplements of minerals, vitamin C, B-vitamins, rhodiola rosea and pregnenolone (with or without DHEA). Occasionally, I use bioidentical cortisol for the short-term to restore any extremely low cortisol levels. Another powerful therapy for adrenal fatigue, and for improving energy, is intravenous nutritional therapy (see Chapter 10).

As for the thyroid, I check for antibodies to determine if there is any autoimmune thyroid disease, and I check the Free T3 and Reverse T3. Free T3 is the active thyroid hormone that helps with metabolism, energy, and to increase body heat. Reverse T3 is a byproduct of T4, and is considered a useless thyroid hormone. I see so many patients with high levels of Reverse T3 and very low levels of Free T3 who were told by an endocrinologist that their thyroid was normal because they had a TSH level of 1.

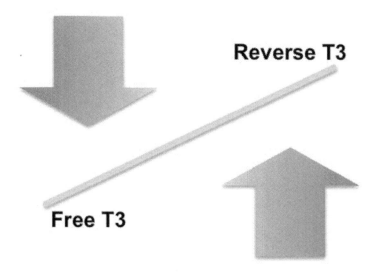

In this situation, where you have more Reverse T3 than Free T3, you will be cold, fat and tired.

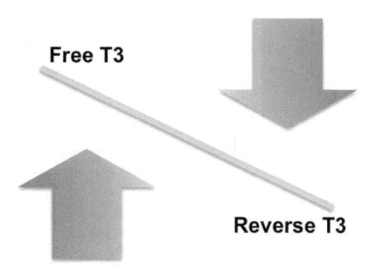

In this situation, where your Free T3 is higher than your Reverse T3, you will have more energy, be warmer and have an easier time losing weight.

"Everyone deserves to live their life
with energy and youthfulness."

While there are many different circumstances and conditions that bring people to Dr. Lee for the wonderful care he provides, my condition began when I was only 27. Due to my younger age, almost everyone I saw in the medical field did not take my symptoms seriously. They said I was too young to be experiencing those symptoms and therefore it must be something else, or that it was nothing more than my imagination.

In my particular situation, the first time I noticed any health concerns was after my daughter was born. My first and primary symptom at the time was anxiety. The old saying, "And I was never the same again," is how I would always describe how I felt. Then, while reading an article one day about hormonal imbalances, and why you are best treated with bioidentical hormones, I knew what I needed to do.

However, the problem was finding a doctor that would listen to me and not just put me on synthetic hormones or birth control, or simply tell me I was experiencing "the symptoms of chronic fatigue." At one particular low point, I became so desperate to feel better that I finally agreed to take birth control pills—despite knowing from before that those pills only made me feel worse.

By the time my daughter was four, my symptoms had worsened drastically. I was having extreme fatigue, headaches, bad acne, mood swings, weight gain, was cold constantly and just did not feel good at all. I started going to a gynecologist who began treating me with bioidentical hormones; however, after six months I still felt bad, was growing excessively tired and was bordering on total desperation and depression as I began thinking that not even bioidentical hormones could help me.

I no longer possessed the strength to get out of bed. I'd stopped going anywhere, and all I wanted to do was sleep. I simply did not have the motivation to see another doctor. But then, my husband came home at lunch one day to find me asleep—and he spent four hours trying to wake me! When I finally awoke, he said that he was taking me to a doctor he'd heard some great things about. It was Dr. Lee.

When I went to see Dr. Lee for the first time, he immediately impressed me with how thorough he was—and still is. He listened to everything that my husband and I had to say. He then looked at my blood work—the same blood so many other doctors had seen—and he immediately recognized a thyroid problem that no one else had seen.

He went on to conclude that I had adrenal fatigue, a hormone imbalance, low vitamin D levels, heavy metal toxicity and a low thyroid. This was the first time in my long journey that we left a doctor's office feeling like there was hope!

Dr. Lee started changing my hormones right away, and soon had me on pregnenolone for my adrenal fatigue. In just a few days I felt a huge difference, but not yet completely back to normal, and then I remembered what Dr. Lee had said: "You didn't get this way in one day so be patient, this is going to be a process." But now, thanks to everything Dr. Lee has done for me, every day I feel as though I take another step toward better health.

So far, Dr. Lee has balanced my hormones, taught me the importance of nutrition and exercise, helped me achieve regular bowel movements, treated my adrenal fatigue and, during the process, brought my cortisol levels back into the normal range.

Furthermore, he supplemented my diet with vitamins and minerals to correct my insufficiencies and calm my anxiety. In addition, he helped me detoxify my body of heavy metal toxicity, prescribed human chorionic gonadotropin to help me lose weight (I've already lost 14 pounds!) and, most recently, he successfully adjusted my thyroid—which vastly improved my quality of life in only five months.

I feel as though Dr. Lee has given me back my life! And that is exactly why I am always encouraging anyone who is suffering from any sort of life-altering symptoms to not wait any longer. Or, to not allow a doctor who doesn't have the proper experience to try and convince you that anything less than your individualized hormonal balance and optimization is the best way to go. Do not settle for less.

Everyone deserves to live their life with energy and youthfulness. Thank you Dr. Lee for making that possible for me.

— Dee Dee Albritton

Before optimizing the thyroid, I will first work on the adrenal fatigue.   I like to explain the reason for this by asking patients to consider their body like a car, where cortisol is the fuel of your body, and the thyroid is their accelerator pedal. Before stepping on the gas pedal, you need to always make sure the car (body) is fueled up (cortisol). The reason for this is that you can "burn out your engine" if the thyroid is treated before addressing the adrenal fatigue.

As for insulin resistance, or having too much insulin, this is a major problem for many people. Everyone needs to understand that if you eat too much sugar (bread, pasta, rice, potatoes, ice cream, cakes, pies, sodas, grapes, oranges, candy or alcohol) then your insulin levels will spike. These high insulin levels will increase the inflammation in the body and lead to many chronic diseases—ranging from obesity to dementia. (See *Your Best Investment: Secrets to a Healthy Body and Mind* to learn more about the dangers of insulin resistance, and to learn about a healthy eating plan.)

Growth hormone replacement is possible therapy for increasing your energy, but only after everything else in your body is balanced/ optimized. Using the body as a car analogy, growth hormone is like turbocharging your engine.   It is waste of time and money to turbocharge your engine if you have four flat tires (adrenal fatigue, low thyroid, low testosterone and insulin resistance).

Because the process of dispensing growth hormone is highly regulated by the United States government, you need to properly qualify for this hormone. The best test for this is an insulin hypoglycemia test, or insulin tolerance test (ITT). I do this test regularly in my office to confirm if there is any adult-onset growth hormone deficiency.

"I finally realized the devastating effects stress and anxiety had on my hormones, and consequently my health."
I am a 25-year-old law school student in Jacksonville, Florida and I drive two-and-a-half hours every week to see Dr. Lee. I initially came to Dr. Lee

because I was concerned about the toll that chronic stress and anxiety had taken on my body.

A saliva test revealed that my symptoms were caused by hormonal imbalances and progesterone deficiency. To correct these imbalances, Dr. Lee started me on bioidentical hormones and nutritional supplements. However, in six months, when Dr. Lee discovered that I also had adrenal fatigue, I finally realized the devastating effects stress and anxiety had on my hormones, and consequently my health. In the six short months that I have been under Dr. Lee's care for hormonal imbalance and adrenal fatigue, my life has turned around. I have more energy, I am sleeping better, I am thinking clearly—I feel like myself again! Not only has Dr. Lee helped me to get my health back, he has helped me to get my life back.

What distinguishes Dr. Lee from other physicians is the handprint he leaves on the hearts of his patients when he touches their lives. Thank you, Dr. Lee, for touching my life, and for showing me the path to health and happiness.

— Allison Kaylor

Gut Health

Leaky gut is an important concept since this can be the cause of many problems. Leaky gut, or intestinal hyperpermeability, is where you have a small or microscopic holes in your small intestine that allow toxins into your blood system. It's like the outside world (which includes your gut, from your mouth to your anus—see Chapter 1) can get into your body (the inside world). Leaky gut is a gateway—a slippery slope—to chronic disease. You seriously need to find out if you have a leaky gut, and there are several tests to determine if you have this condition.

To confirm a leaky gut, I prefer the lactulose mannitol test, or the antibodies to zonulin test. Zonulin is the protein that regulates the "tight junctions" of your gut wall. Zonulin is what opens those billions of gateway spaces between those billions of cells, allowing some substances to pass through, while keeping harmful bacteria and toxins out. Zonulin is produced in the gut, and if it is elevated, then the tight junctures of your gut will open up even more—allowing harmful bacteria and toxins to pass through. Unfortunately, checking strictly for zonulin levels is limited to research only, and is not yet commercially available.

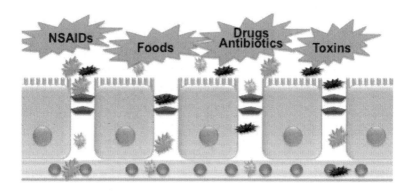

Causes of leaky gut may include: NSAIDs (non-steroidal anti-inflammatory drugs), certain foods, drugs, antibiotics and toxins. Then, as depicted above, a leaky gut will allow these larger molecules to leak into the blood system.

If you are diagnosed with a leaky gut, then this can be the cause of your low energy (since a leaky gut causes poor absorption of nutrients). With a leaky gut, toxins or microorganisms like bacteria, yeast and fungus can enter your blood system. These microorganisms can then compete for the nutrients that your body needs. Not everyone in my roster of patients has leaky gut, but I would conservatively estimate that about half of my patients have some degree of a leaky gut.

Treatment of leaky gut is best accomplished through the 4R Program: remove the offending agent, replace with digestive enzymes, reinoculate with probiotics, and repair with glutamine. For details on the 4R Program, and more about leaky gut, see Chapter 1.

Liver Detox

Another important concept on how best to obtain better energy is to detoxify better. Your liver does many important functions, but one of the most important is to alter the fat-soluble toxins so they can be safely eliminated. If all toxins were water-soluble then you could just urinate them out, but they are not, and this is where your liver steps in.

The analogy I like to tell my patients is that your liver is like a barrel with a spigot. If your spigot is not wide open, or if you overfill your barrel with too many toxins, then your barrel will overflow. The toxins that your body needs to get rid of on a daily basis are: pesticides, herbicides, perfumes, cosmetic makeup, lipstick, deodorant, fumes (such as pumping gasoline), PBAs (from plastic containers, such as water bottles), radiation, processed foods and the thousands of chemicals that pollute the air and water.

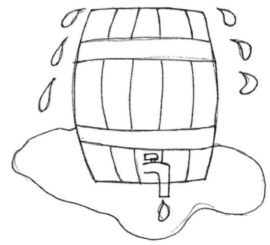

As explained in Chapter 11, this "liver" is overflowing with toxins. It needs a liver detox, or it will overflow toxins and free radicals into your body, which will damage the most important structure in your body—your DNA. Before that happens, the key is to "open the spigot" by doing a liver detox. It is never too late to do a liver detox—even if your "barrel" is already overflowing.

Artwork by Connor Lee (nine years old).

The spigot represents your body's ability to get rid of those toxins, and if you take in more than your spigot can get rid of, then your body is due to fail. The barrel will overflow with toxins and these toxins can then be stored in your fat, or in your brain. These accumulated toxins can cause chronic inflammation and damage your DNA, which can lead to chronic disease, tiredness, developmental disorders, neurotoxicity and cancer.

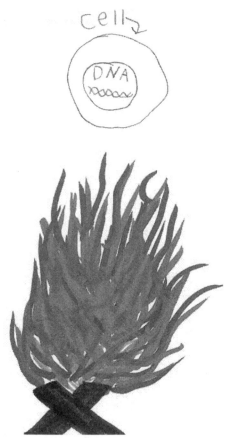

This illustration represents chronic inflammation as a fire that is damaging to DNA. Damaged DNA causes premature aging, chronic disease, cancer and early death.

Artwork by Connor Lee (nine years old) and Nathan Lee (eight years old).

The best way to open up your spigot all the way (maximize your body's ability to get rid of toxins) is to improve the different routes of elimination available to your body—like through your kidneys, skin (sweating), liver and daily bowel movements. In addition, hormonal balance, exercise, laughter, vitamins, proper nutrition, minerals, enzymes, amino acids and antioxidants will help your energy significantly. And, most of my patients have had positive results with a medical food we offer as part of my ten-day liver detox program.

Intravenous Nutrition

Overall, the ultimate therapy is intravenous therapy, which guarantees absorption and brings the essential vitamins, minerals and especially glutathione (needed for phase I and phase II for the liver to detoxify) into your cells where they can then do their jobs of: lowering inflammation, lowering oxidative stress, removing toxins from the cells and supporting the mitochondria to make energy. This approach will definitively help to reverse your tiredness, while helping you to achieve optimal health.

"I had resigned myself to the belief that at my age,
you're supposed to feel old and tired."

The trip I took to Orlando and the Institute for Hormonal Balance became a milestone in my life. Dr. Lee found my testosterone level to be extremely low and my estrogen level high—which I'm now convinced is a condition in a lot of older men that isn't recognized by most physicians.

With Dr. Lee's care and supplements, my atrial fibrillation has been rectified. At 63 I now have a steady heartbeat, no weight problems, an abundance of energy and I'm sleeping better and feeling better than I did 20 or even 30 years ago!

Until Dr. Lee, I had resigned myself to the belief that at my age, you're supposed to feel old and tired all the time—along with the little aches, pains and a tremor in my right hand. How wrong I was! Thanks to Dr. Lee my life has changed dramatically. He is intelligent, caring and has your best interest at heart—and it's obvious that he definitely practices what he preaches. I don't feel like a simple "thank you" could ever be enough for what Dr. Lee has accomplished with my health.

I've been lucky enough to make a few right decisions in my life, but seeing Dr. Lee is one of my best decisions. I thank him from the bottom of my heart.

— Darlow "Rex" Rexroat

P.S. The best gift you can ever give your body is a trip to see Dr. Lee!

Remember, chronic inflammation is the main source of tiredness and chronic diseases, and the main source of inflammation is from leaky gut syndrome. The leaky gut syndrome is usually from a delayed food sensitivity or food intolerance that is IgG mediated (certain class of antibody that is involved in the immune system). It is crucial that you have a healthy gut in order to digest and absorb the foods you eat in order to provide the proper nutrients to your cells. Also, a key step in reversing tiredness and reducing chronic inflammation is to balance the hormones with bioidentical hormones. Hormonal balance involves addressing adrenal fatigue and then addressing the other hormones, like the sex hormones, and optimizing the thyroid. The last hormone that should be addressed is the growth hormone, which is like turbocharging. I often tell my patients that if you want to turbocharge your car, then you need to fix your four flat tires first.

Other Considerations

Other important issues that help with energy production and reversing tiredness are: detoxifying the toxins in your body, exercising regularly, sleeping seven to eight hours every night and quitting smoking. It is also crucial to have daily bowel movements to help with the detoxification process so that the metabolic waste and toxins do not reenter back into your body's circulation.

It is also important to note that there are prescription medications that can be causing your tiredness. Cholesterol lowering medications called statins—such as Lipitor®, Crestor® and Zocor®—can all lower coenzyme Q-10 (CoQ-10) or ubiquinone levels. These cholesterol medications are one of the most prescribed medications on the market, and have been shown to lower CoQ-10 levels by 40 percent.[1-2] CoQ-10 is crucial to the energy production in the mitochondria of each and every cell in your body.

If any of my patients is on a statin therapy, then I recommend the use of CoQ-10 with it. Other medications that can lower CoQ-10 levels are certain beta-blockers, a class of blood pressure medication and hydrochlorothiazide, which is another class of blood pressure medications.[3-4] So, for all of my tired patients, I often recommend an extra supplement of CoQ-10—often in its liquid version for better absorption.

"I've found the energy to come out of retirement."

I am a 71-year-old physician and have been with Dr. Lee for many years. Dr. Lee has helped me by increasing my energy, by reducing my four blood pressure medications down to two, and by losing 30 pounds. Dr. Lee has optimized my testosterone, growth hormone and my nutrition.

I have also received several detox treatments in his office and I've noticed that I tend to focus better after the treatments.

I'm now enjoying life more and, thanks to Dr. Lee, I've found the energy to come out of retirement and return to part time work as a physician again.

— Dean Shull Jr. M.D.

Energy Supplements

To help reverse tiredness, there are four supplements I like to give my patients. One is a combination pill (Prob-Zyme) that has digestive enzymes and probiotics. The other three are: CoQ-10 (100 to 300 mg a day); a drink called Power Fuel that has D-Ribose and Acetyl L-Carnitine; and a supplement with DMG (Dimethylglycine). A little history on DMG is that it was referred to as vitamin B15 when first discovered as pangamic acid in 1951; however, it is no longer considered a vitamin by strict definition of the word.

I like to call DMG by the nickname "Damn Mighty Good" since it has helped many of my patients with their low energy. Damn Mighty Good (DMG) has also been shown to improve performance in athletes.[5] DMG helps you make glutathione, which is needed in your liver to help detoxify any toxins that are damaging your DNA. DMG also helps by donating a methyl group (CH3, a carbon molecule attached with 3 hydrogen molecules), which is known as methylation. Methylation is a biochemical process essential to life, and is part of the phase II of detoxification in the liver. Methylation also adds a methyl group to other substances that depend on methyl groups to complete their synthesis—such as vitamins, hormones, enzymes, DNA and neurotransmitters.

By combining these energy production supplements with nutrition and absorption supplements—such as vitamin D3, omega 3 and a good multivitamin—your potential for optimizing energy production will increase. As a guideline, typical doses for these supplements are given in a chart at the end of this chapter. (The doses are provided as a guideline. Your recommended usage and doses may vary.)

So, as you now know, the good news is that you can reverse tiredness—but it does take work. First, it is critical to reduce chronic inflammation so that it does not lead to oxidative stress or to the production of toxic chemicals (free radicals) that can damage your cells, DNA and decrease your energy.

In summary, to produce more energy, which comes from your mitochondria (the energy source of your cells), you have to eat healthy (more vegetables and fiber), do regular physical activity, add extra digestive enzymes and probiotics to your diet, and add nutritional support with vitamins, antioxidants, minerals and amino acids. The most effective way to improve your energy is intravenous nutritional therapy. (See Chapter 10 to learn more about intravenous nutrition.)

It is crucial that you have a healthy gut to digest and absorb the foods you eat in order to provide the proper nutrients to our cells. Also, you must balance your hormones with bioidentical hormones, sleep seven to eight hours a night, laugh more, reduce stress, quit smoking and detoxify the toxins. By taking all these steps you will reverse tiredness.

Increasing Energy Production Through Supplements
Optimizing energy production through a balanced combination of energy, nutrition and absorption supplements

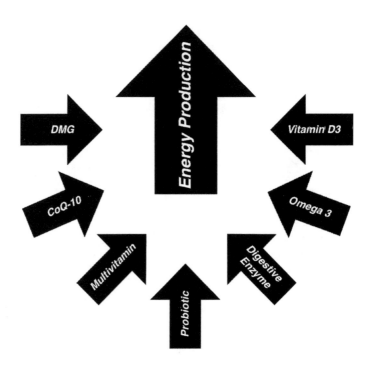

Dimethylglycine (DMG) — 100 to 500 mg daily
CoQ-10 — 100 to 300 mg daily
Multivitamin/Multimineral — 2 to 8 pills daily
Probiotic — 3 to 5 billion microorganisms daily
Digestive Enzyme — 1 to 3 pills daily
Omega-3 — 2 to 4 grams daily
Vitamin D3 — 2000 to 5000 units daily

This chart is intended only as a guideline.
Recommendations and doses may vary from person to person.

CHAPTER 15 REVIEW

— While there is no magic pill for reversing tiredness, I often focus on hormonal balance, gut health, liver detox, better sleep, and better nutrition.

— Eat organic foods and avoid any processed foods with chemicals such as: pesticides, fertilizers, fungicides, herbicides, antibiotics, hormones or preservatives.

— Keep your blood sugars under control by avoiding any artificial sweeteners and refined carbohydrates like: white bread, white pasta, white potatoes, white rice or foods with high fructose corn syrup that will cause a spike in your insulin.

— Carbohydrates from vegetables are an excellent source of: fiber, minerals, vitamins and phytonutrients.

— As an easy to remember guideline, I recommend consuming different colors of vegetables (two to three servings) with each meal. This will help to maximize the power of the antioxidants from each unique vegetable.

— Consume four grams a day of omega-3 from a healthy source such as: walnuts, olive oil, flax seed, winter squash, fish, soy and bean, just to name a few.

— For protein, lean meats that were grass fed—not grain-fed—and were raised free-range are recommended.

— Leaky gut, or intestinal hyperpermeability, is where you have a small or microscopic hole in the small intestine that allows toxins into your blood system. Leaky gut is a gateway—a slippery slope—to chronic disease.

— It is crucial that you have a healthy gut in order to digest and absorb the foods you eat in order to provide proper nutrients to your cells.

— Some common supplements that can help with energy are: CoQ-10 (100 mg to 300 mg a day), vitamin D3 (2000 to 5000 units a day), Dimethylglycine (DMG 500 mg a day), probiotics, digestive enzymes, omega 3, multivitamins and multi-minerals.

CONCLUSION

I'm Not Tired Anymore!

Even as you're living the healthiest life possible, harmful things (pollution and stress, for example) will still find their way into your life. The difference now is that you're prepared to fight back with a well-balanced arsenal. Such balance is best achieved by diversification.

In much the same way that financial wealth is achieved by diversification, your optimal health is best achieved by diversification —investing in a combination of exercise, diet, hormonal balance, nutritional support, sleep and, when needed, intravenous vitamins and detoxification.

Do It With Passion and a Sense of Wonder!

So now you have it. The knowledge to feel good, have more energy and look younger—when put to use—is your gateway to leading a healthier and better life. It's the basis of my practice, the core things I teach and share with my patients every day. The ultimate goal of optimizing your hormones, detoxing, having a healthy gut and nutritional support is to protect the most precious structure in your body: your DNA.

We live in a toxic world these days, with increasingly more chemicals being produced that pollute our environment.   And, we are experiencing increases in: diabetes, obesity, autoimmune disease, neurodegenerative disease, heart disease, and cancer. Now, more than ever, to live life to the fullest, you must optimize your hormones, detoxify, for a healthy gut, lead an active lifestyle with daily exercise, eat less sugar, eat more vegetables and fiber, and include nutritional supplements in your diet.

However, as I wrote this book, I began to realize that my patients were teaching me something as well. During the lengthy process of translating my work onto these pages, I began to see a consistent pattern. The patients responding best to treatment—thriving on the new life they're earning—these are the people who approach life with passion and a sense of wonder. It's something that goes beyond the positive attitude, which, of course, is important as well.

I love the tagline from Beachbody®, which is, "Decide. Commit. Succeed." Decide to be healthy, commit to work out and eat healthy and to do whatever it takes and you will succeed in having a healthy body and mind. In my practice most people that voluntarily come in to see me have already decided that they need some extra help and guidance, and they have decided that they want to get their youth and energy back. The hardest thing in life is the "C" word, and that is commitment. I originally thought commitment was a man's weakness (to marriage), but I see so many women that just don't want to commit to exercise, or to change their lifestyle (such as drinking wine every night), or even commit to a ten-day liver cleanse to help their liver detox. It does take passion <u>and</u> commitment.

The commitment phrase I like best came from the famous Florida quarterback, Tim Tebow, when he said, "Hard work beats talent when talent doesn't work hard." Another way I have heard it said is, "Hard work trumps talent." I often say that to my young boys—while pointing out that it takes work in life to succeed.

Sometimes, I make my boys walk the golf course, instead of riding the cart, when we play a round of golf. I truly believe you have to suffer a little in life to accomplish anything. That's why I love the challenges of hiking, kayaking, cycling and exploring new places in this world. And, true to that phrase, my friends and I usually suffer through some body aches after we do those adventures. Whenever you start to exercise, you will have some discomfort, but think of it as a little reward. It will get better each time you do it. Trust me.

It will always be easier to take the path of least resistance, but that does not make it the best path. Even though it might feel wonderful to eat and drink whatever you wanted, and never have to exercise to stay healthy, the truth is that we are not created to live such a lifestyle. Our ancestors were hunters and gatherers. They had to find food every day in order to survive, which meant they had to take care of their bodies in order to hunt and gather. Unfortunately, most of our society has lost that priority in life—the priority to take care of your body in order to survive. And now, more and more, I see this downfall in other countries when I travel around the world.

It is unfortunate that when we have our youth we pursue wealth, but after we accumulate some wealth, then we spend it on our health—when all along, the true wealth is always our health.

You can have all the wealth in the world but you can never buy health. You need to earn it. So commit to being healthy and exercise regularly.

For some reason, when I go to many social functions lately, the first thing people say to me, even though I may never have met them (but they know of me), is that they don't think they exercise enough. I don't know why they say this when I first meet them. Maybe it's a subconscious guilt thing. Whatever it is, some people are simply lazy and overweight. They would rather take a pill than exercise. These are my most challenging patients.

For example, if I advised one of these patients to get a Vo2 Max test to receive a customized, high-intensity 20-minute anaerobic workout that is guaranteed to help them to lose weight (see Chapter 12), they might give me an excuse like, "I want to check out this new fad workout that will probably not do anything," or say, "My schedule is too busy for a Vo2 Max test." Unfortunately, these patients are neglecting the most important part of their health, and that is to be physically fit. This is why there are some days I find myself wishing there was a pill for reversing laziness.

Bottom line, for those who neglect their health, or don't want to be physically fit and would rather take the path of least resistance, then they will most likely regret it. After having their debilitating stroke, or suffering from a heart attack, then maybe they will begin spending some of their wealth to achieve health. What they don't realize though, is that while it is true that you are never too old to become healthy, it does become harder the longer you wait to start.

However, for those who are overweight with other chronic issues (such as joint pain, diabetes, high blood pressure, high cholesterol, etc.), their body is like a ticking time bomb, ready to explode. Their chronic inflammation and high insulin levels, combined with nutritional deficiencies and a liver that does not detox well enough, are creating the perfect storm—a storm that will damage their DNA. Then, once their DNA is damaged, chronic disease (stroke, heart attack, diabetes, etc.), premature aging, cancer and death will soon follow. Sadly, I see this condition daily in my practice. The good news is that a body can recover, if it is given the right nutrition and hormones.

Oprah hit the nail on the head when she said, "Passion is energy. Feel the power that comes from focusing on what excites you." I am thankful that every day, I get to focus on helping people regain the energy to pursue their passions.

Get Out There and Enjoy Life!

So, now that you're living healthier and enjoying more energy, reward yourself by doing more—get out there and enjoy life more! There is so much to explore and enjoy in the world when you can truly say, "I feel good, and I look younger."

Appendix: Inflammation

NFKB

The keystone of inflammation is a protein complex called nuclear factor kappa beta (NFKB). It plays a critical role in infection, cancer, inflammation and autoimmune disease. NFKB are present in cells and are known as the first responders to a toxic stimulus. Chemicals called cytokines activate NFKB and then, once activated, the NFKB turn on other enzymes like cyclooxygenase and lipoxygenase. These cascading events then lead to the production of harmful eicosanoid hormones like thromboxanes A2, Leukotriene B4 and prostaglandin—which then cause clotting, more inflammation and fever. Again, NFKB is a first responder and once activated it will call for backup, which can only lead to further damage.

There are many events that can trigger an increase of NFKB. Some examples include stress, infection, depression, high glucose, environmental pollution, toxins, obesity, high fat diet, smoking and high homocysteine. (Elevated blood levels of the sulfur-containing amino acid, homocysteine, have been linked to an increased risk of premature coronary artery disease, stroke and venous blood clots, even among people who have normal cholesterol levels). All of these conditions can turn on inflammatory cytokines, which activate NFKB, which then turns on the chronic inflammation.

From there, many diseases are associated with activated NFKB, such as type 1 diabetes, type 2 diabetes, high cholesterol, atherosclerosis, heart disease, stroke, lung disease, Crohn's disease, glaucoma, AIDS, Parkinson disease, inflammatory bowel disease and cancer, just to name a few.

Cytokines

The markers for inflammation are called cytokines, which can be measured in your blood. Cytokines are the signaling molecules used by your cells to communicate with each other. For example, cytokines such as interleukin-6 (IL-6) or tumor necrosis factor alpha (TNF-alpha) will turn on NFKB, which then turn on chronic inflammation.

The Framingham Heart Study showed that an increase in IL-6 and TNF-alpha indicates a shortened lifespan.[1] In addition, a geriatric study found that there was nearly a nine-fold increase in mortality with an increase of IL-6.[2] Cancer studies have shown that there is a correlation between high levels of TNF-alpha and a poor prognosis.[3] Another clinical arena in which cytokines can indicate higher mortality is heart failure. In fact, high levels of IL-6 and TNF-alpha have been strongly associated with increased mortality in chronic heart failure patients.[4]

Measuring Inflammation

While there are many different tests to measure inflammation, I like to measure C-reactive protein (CRP) because the test is relatively inexpensive, and it is a great marker for heart disease. I usually measure CRP (with a blood test) in all my patients over the age of 35. Another inexpensive blood marker for inflammation is the ESR (erythrocyte sedimentation rate); however, the ESR is more of a primitive test when it comes to checking for inflammation.

Another test that that I like to use is the AA/EPA ratio (arachidonic acid to eicosapentaenoic acid ratio), which is a more sophisticated way to measure systemic inflammation. This is a blood test that compares your "good" fatty acids (omega-3) to your "bad" fatty acids (omega-6). The higher the number you have, the higher your risk for developing chronic disease. If you have too low of a number, then you're at risk for having a weak immune system—or, in other words, you may be prone to more infections. Genova Diagnostics® or Metametrix™ can run this test. It is a more expensive test, but very useful.

Now, my favorite test to see how well your body is doing is to measure if you have cell membrane damage, or DNA damage, by measuring lipid peroxide tests for cell membrane damage or measuring 8-OHdG (8-hydroxydeoxyguanosine) for DNA damage. Although you could measure for other cytokines, like IL-6 and TNF, or for other interleukins, I prefer to measure if you have cell membrane damage or DNA damage—which, I believe, is the more important information.

GLOSSARY

A

acromegaly—Hormonal disorder where the pituitary gland produces excess amounts of growth hormone.

ACTH (adrenocorticotropic hormone)—Hormone that is produced from the anterior pituitary gland that stimulates the adrenal glands to release cortisol. An ACTH-secreting pituitary adenoma is one of the causes of Cushing's syndrome, which, is characterized by excess cortisol production. ACTH deficiency results in low cortisol levels and adrenal insufficiency, which can be life threatening.

ACTH stimulation test—Laboratory stimulation test that checks the response of cortisol levels in order to diagnosis adrenal insufficiency.

Addison's disease—Disease where the adrenal glands do not make enough cortisol and/or aldosterone (salt hormone). There are different causes of Addison's disease, such as an autoimmune cause of Addison's disease, which is when the body's immune system attacks and destroys the adrenal glands.

adrenal cortex—Outer portion of the adrenal gland which produces cortisol, which regulate carbohydrate and fat metabolism, and aldosterone (salt) hormones, which regulate salt and water balance in the body. The deepest layer of the adrenal cortex makes the sex hormone DHEA.

adrenal fatigue—Condition where the adrenal glands do not make enough cortisol and/or DHEA and/or aldosterone (adrenal hormones).

adrenal glands—Triangle-shaped glands that sit on top of the kidneys and regulate stress response through the synthesis of hormones which include cortisol, DHEA, aldosterone (salt hormone) and adrenaline.

adrenal hormone—The four major hormones made by the adrenal gland: cortisol, aldosterone, DHEA and adrenaline.

adrenal insufficiency—See adrenal fatigue.

adrenocorticotropic hormone—See ACTH.

ALA (alpha-linolenic acid)—Type of omega-3 fatty acid found in plants. Similar to the omega-3 fatty acids that are in fish oil (eicosapentaenoic acid, or EPA, and docosahexaenoic acid, or DHA) and can be converted into EPA and DHA in the body. Is highly concentrated in flaxseed oil and, to a lesser extent, in canola, soy, perilla, and walnut oils. (Not to be confused with alpha-lipoic acid, which may sometimes be called ALA as well.)

albumin—An important protein that carries hormones, drugs and electrolytes in the circulation.

aldosterone—An adrenal hormone (salt hormone or mineralocorticoid hormone) that helps a person's body keep nutrients, such as sodium and potassium, in balance.

alpha-linolenic acid—See ALA. (Not to be confused with alpha-lipoic acid, which may sometimes be called ALA as well.)

alpha-lipoic acid—Universal antioxidant for energy production, blood sugar regulation and the maintenance of a healthy neural system. Helps reduce the complications associated with diabetes, such as pain and numbness. Has the ability to neutralize many different types of free-radicals, and provides a broad spectrum of support to the body's antioxidant network. (Not to be confused with alpha-linolenic acid, which may sometimes be called ALA as well.)

androgens—Hormones that help to develop sex organs in men, as well as contribute to sexual functions in men and women.

andropause—Biological change characterized by a gradual decline in androgens and experienced by men during, and after, mid-life.

antiandrogens—Substances that inhibit the biological effects of androgenic hormones.

antidiuretic hormone—Secreted by the posterior pituitary gland to regulate the amount of water excreted by the kidneys.

apoptosis—Process of programmed cell death that occurs in multicellular organisms. Biochemical events lead to characteristic cell changes and then death.

B

benign prostatic hyperplasia (enlarged prostate)—non-cancerous enlargement of the prostate gland, a common occurrence in older men.

bioavailable testosterone—Represents the fraction of circulating testosterone that readily enters cells and better reflects the bioactivity of testosterone than does the measurement of serum total testosterone.

bioidentical hormones—Compounds that have exactly the same chemical and molecular structure as hormones that are produced in the human body.

BMD (bone mineral density)—Test to measure the density of minerals (such as calcium) in bones using a special X-ray, which is then interpreted to estimate the strength of bones. Bone mineral density is measured to see if one has bone loss.

BMI (body mass index)—Derived from the weight and height of a person, a BMI above 30 will usually reveal obesity; although, weight lifters with more muscle and lower amounts of body fat may also have a BMI over 30.

body mass index—See BMI.

bone mineral density—see BMD.

C

C-reactive protein (CRP)—Protein found in the blood that is elevated in response to inflammation. It is made in the liver and is a marker for inflammation. (CRP is not to be confused with C- peptide.)

calcitonin—Protein hormone secreted by cells in the thyroid gland to inhibit bone degradation and stimulate the uptake of calcium and phosphate by bones.

celiac disease (gluten sensitive enteropathy)—Digestive disease that damages the small intestine because of a sensitivity to gluten, which is found in wheat, rye, barley, and oats. This hereditary disorder interferes with the absorption of nutrients from food.

cholesterol—White crystalline substance found in animal tissues and various foods that is normally synthesized by the liver, and is an important constituent of cell membranes as well as a precursor to steroid hormones.

chronic inflammation—Leads to a progressive shift in the type of cells which are present at the site of inflammation and is characterized by the simultaneous destruction and healing of the tissue from the inflammatory process. Without inflammation, wounds and infections would never heal and progressive destruction of the tissue would compromise survival; however, chronic inflammation can also lead to a host of diseases.

congenital adrenal hyperplasia (CAH)—Group of inherited adrenal gland disorders that does not produce enough of the hormones cortisol and aldosterone; but produces too much androgen. Infants born with CAH may be born with ambiguous genitalia, which could make it difficult to determine if they are male or female. Approximately 95 percent of CAH cases are due to 21-hydroxylase deficiency.

corticotropin releasing hormone (CRH)—Hormone produced by the hypothalamus that stimulates the anterior pituitary gland to release adrenocorticotropic hormone (ACTH).

cortisol—Hormone produced by the adrenal gland which is involved in the stress response, reduces inflammation, opposes insulin so it increases glucose, and aids in fat and protein metabolism.

CRH—See corticotropin releasing hormone.

Crohn's Disease—Inflammatory disease of the intestines that may affect any part, from the mouth to the anus. It can cause belly pain, diarrhea, bloody stool, vomiting or weight loss. It is an autoimmune disease in which the body's immune system attacks the intestines causing inflammation.

CRP—See C-reactive protein.

Cushing's syndrome (hypercortisolism)—Hormonal disorder caused by prolonged exposure of the body's tissues to high levels of the hormone cortisol.

cytokines—Any of various protein molecules secreted by cells of the immune system that serve to regulate the immune system.

D

dehydroepiandrosterone (DHEA)—Steroid hormone produced by the adrenal glands that helps build up muscle, improves memory and helps with vitality.

delayed food sensitivity (food intolerance)—Adverse responses to specific food(s) or food ingredient(s). Delayed allergic reactions, which are mediated by IgG, are different from a true food allergy that is mediated by IgE. Symptoms from delayed food sensitivity include chronic stuffy nose, chronic sinusitis, bad breath, tiredness, cough and headaches.

DHA (docosahexaenoic acid)—As part of omega-3, DHA is a major fatty acid in sperm and the retina. Low levels of DHA have been associated with Alzheimer's disease.

DHEA—See dehydroepiandrosterone.

diabetes—Disease in which blood glucose levels are above normal. The body of a person with diabetes either doesn't make enough insulin or can't use its own insulin as well as it should.

dihydrotestosterone—Male hormone that is more potent than testosterone, and is converted from testosterone within the prostate.

dimethylglycine (DMG or pangamic acid)—A derivative of the amino acid glycine that, when first discovered, was called vitamin B15; but, is no longer considered a vitamin. DMG helps make glutathione, which is needed in the liver to help detoxify any toxins that are damaging DNA. DMG also helps by donating a methyl group (CH3, a carbon molecule attached with 3 hydrogen molecules), which is known as methylation. Methylation is a biochemical process essential to life, and is part of the phase II of detoxification in the liver. Methylation also adds a methyl group to other substances (such as vitamins, hormones, enzymes, DNA and neurotransmitters) that depend on methyl groups to complete their synthesis.

DMG—See dimethylglycine.

Docosahexaenoic acid—See DHA.

E

eicosapentaenoic acid (EPA)—Found in fish oils, especially from salmon and other cold-water fish, and acts to lower inflammation in the blood.   EPA and docosahexaenoic acid (DHA) are the two principal omega-3 fatty acids.   The body has a limited ability to manufacture EPA and DHA by converting alpha-linolenic acid (ALA), which is found in flaxseed oil, canola oil or walnuts.

endocrine disruptor—Natural and man-made chemicals that can either mimic or disrupt the action of hormones.

endocrinologist—Medical doctor that has done extra training in the field of hormones. Endocrinologists are specialists in diabetes, thyroid disease, thyroid nodules, thyroid cancer, calcium disorders, sodium disorders, short stature, growth hormone disorders, adrenal diseases, osteoporosis, and pituitary problems.

enlarged prostate—See benign prostatic hyperplasia.

EPA—See eicosapentaenoic acid.

estradiol—As a type of estrogen, it is a female sex hormone produced mainly by the ovaries and is responsible for growth of breast tissue, maturation of long bones, and development of the secondary sexual characteristics. It is the estrogen of youth.

estriol—Type of estrogen produced mainly during pregnancy. Estriol has been shown to protect women from breast cancer.

estrogen—Group of steroid compounds that are the primary female sex hormones. They promote the development of female secondary sex characteristics and control aspects of regulating the menstrual cycle.

estrogen therapy (ET)—Hormone therapy treatment in which women take estrogen orally, transdermally or vaginally to treat certain symptoms of menopause. It is not advised to take estrogen by mouth since it can increase the risk for heart disease and stroke.

estrone—Type of estrogen that is mainly produced during menopause. High levels of estrone has been associated with breast cancer. Premarin® has estrone in it.

ET—See estrogen therapy.

F

food allergy—Reaction to the ingestion of a food that causes adverse effects when the immune system does not recognize as safe a protein component (the allergen) of the food to which the individual is sensitive (such as some proteins in peanuts). The immune system then typically produces immunoglobulin E (IgE) antibodies to the allergen, which trigger other cells to release substances that cause inflammation. Allergic reactions are usually localized to a particular part of the body, and symptoms may include asthma, eczema, flushing, and swelling of tissues (such as the lips) or difficulty in breathing. A severe reaction may result in anaphylaxis (as with severe peanut allergy), in which there is a rapid fall in blood pressure and severe shock. Allergic reactions to foods vary in severity and can be potentially fatal.

food intolerance—See delayed food sensitivity.

free radicals—Molecule produced in the body that is necessary for life, such as destroying bacteria. Too much free radical production has been shown to cause DNA damage, which is not desirable. Vitamin A, vitamin E and vitamin C are antioxidants that can reduce free radicals.

free testosterone—Testosterone in the body that is biologically active and unbound to other molecules in the body, such as sex hormone binding globulin.

follicle stimulating hormone (FSH)—In women, FSH helps control the menstrual cycle and the production of eggs by the ovaries. The amount of FSH varies throughout a woman's menstrual cycle and is highest just before she ovulates. FSH is elevated in women with ovarian failure or women in menopause. In men, FSH helps with the production of sperm.

FSH—See follicle stimulating hormone.

G

genetic testing—Tests on blood and other tissue to find genetic disorders.

gland—Organ that synthesizes a substance for release, such as hormones, often into the bloodstream (endocrine gland). An example of an endocrine gland is the thyroid gland that is found in the front of the neck and produces thyroxine (T4), triiodothyronine (T3) and calcitonin hormones.

glucagon—Hormone involved in carbohydrate metabolism or producing more glucose. Produced by the pancreas, it is released when the glucose level in the blood is low (hypoglycemia), causing the liver to convert stored glycogen into glucose and release it into the bloodstream. Glucagon levels are very high in diabetes.

gluten—Consisting of two proteins, gliadin and glutenin, gluten is found in wheat, rye and barley. Gluten is used in the food industry to help make baked food products chewier. Gluten is also used as a food stabilizing agent, and may be found in ketchup and ice cream.

gluten sensitive enteropathy—See celiac disease.

GnRH (gonadotropin releasing hormone)—Also known as luteinizing-hormone releasing hormone (LHRH), this peptide hormone is responsible for the release of gonadotropin (LH and FSH) from the anterior pituitary. GnRH is synthesized and released by the hypothalamus (an upper part of the brain).

gonads—Organ that makes gametes (sperm and egg cells). The gonads in males are the testes and the gonads in females are the ovaries.

gonadotropin—Hormone that stimulate the growth and activity of the gonads, especially any of several pituitary hormones that stimulate the function of the ovaries and testes.

gonadotropin releasing hormone—See GnRH.

glycemia—The concentration of glucose in the blood.

Graves' disease—Most common form of hyperthyroidism, it occurs when the immune system mistakenly attacks the thyroid gland and causes it to overproduce the hormone thyroxine.

growth hormone—Secreted by the pituitary gland, it stimulates growth of bone and, essentially, all tissues of the body by building protein and breaking down fat to provide energy.

gynecomastia—Development of abnormally large mammary glands (breast tissue) in males resulting in breast enlargement.

H

Hashimoto's thyroiditis—The most common cause of underactive thyroid disease, it is an autoimmune condition in which the immune system destroys the thyroid.

heavy metal toxicity—Condition where one has been exposed to a metal either by breathing, swallowing or skin exposure. Common heavy metal toxicity includes mercury, lead, cadmium and arsenic. Heavy metal toxicity is damaging to the body and needs to be removed from the body by chelation.

HGH (human growth hormone)—growth hormone that is mainly used to help children of short stature and also for adults with adult growth hormone deficiency. HGH is an injection that needs to be taken daily.

hirsutism—Excessive growth of thick dark hair in locations where hair growth in women usually is minimal or absent but typical in men, such as the face or chest.

hormone—Made by endocrine glands, hormones are chemical messengers that travel in the bloodstream to tissues or organs. They affect many processes, including growth, metabolism, sexual function, reproduction and mood.

hormone therapy—The use of hormones in medical treatment, such as thyroid hormone replacement for thyroid deficiency.

hot flashes—Sudden wave of mild or intense body heat caused by dilation of capillaries in the skin resulting from decreased levels of estrogen.

HPA (hypothalamic pituitary adrenal axis)—The interaction between the hypothalamus, pituitary and adrenal glands. For example, CRH is released from the hypothalamus gland and CRH stimulates the pituitary gland to secrete ACTH. ACTH then stimulates the adrenal glands to produce cortisol. Later cortisol can inhibit the production of CRH from the hypothalamus gland.

human growth hormone—See HGH.

hydrocortisone—Steroid medication that is similar to cortisol. Hydrocortisone is used in patients with adrenal insufficiency, and also used to treat arthritis and also inflammation.

hypercortisolism— See Cushing's syndrome.

hypoglycemia (low blood sugar)—Occurs when the blood glucose level drops too low to provide enough energy for the body's activities.

hypogonadism—Condition in which the production of sex hormones and germ cells (sperm and eggs) is inadequate. In men it is a condition of low testosterone level, which is considered a lethal disease. In women it is a condition of low estrogen, progesterone and low, or no production, of eggs.

hypothalamic pituitary adrenal axis—See HPA.

hypothalamus—An area of the brain, situated above the pituitary gland, with the important function of connecting the nervous system to the endocrine system via the pituitary gland. The hypothalamus regulates vital autonomic centers and produces hormones that control thirst, hunger, body temperature, sleep, moods, sex drive and the release of hormones—primarily through the pituitary gland.

hypothyroidism—Condition where the thyroid does not produce adequate thyroid hormone. A very common complaint of patients with hypothyroidism is that they are tired and also cold.

I

ICD (International Classification of Diseases and Related Health Problems)—List of codes to classify diseases, including signs, symptoms, abnormal findings, social circumstances, complaints and external causes of injury or disease. ICD is published by the World Health Organization and is made to promote international comparability. The current edition is ICD-10 and the next one, ICD-11, is planned for 2015.

IgE—Certain class of antibody that has an important role against allergies and parasite infections.

IGF-1 (insulin-like growth factor-1)—Protein hormone similar in molecular structure to insulin. Secreted from the liver, it plays an important role in childhood growth and continues to have anabolic effects in adults. Also, it is used to screen for growth hormone deficiency.

IgG—Certain class of antibody that is involved in the secondary immune response. The initial response is IgM (another class of antibody). IgG is involved in delayed food sensitivity.

inflammation—Biological response for the body to heal. Without inflammation wounds and infections would never heal or get rid of infection. Inflammation is a complex reaction which involves many different cytokines.

insulin—A protein pancreatic hormone secreted by the beta cells of the islets of Langerhans that is especially essential for the metabolism of carbohydrates and the regulation of glucose levels in the blood; and, when insufficiently produced, results in diabetes mellitus.

insulin sensitizers—These make cells more responsive to insulin and are commonly used in patients with type 2 diabetes.

insulin-like growth factor-1—See IGF-1.

interleukin—A protein or cytokine that is involved in the immune system and with inflammation. While there are many different interleukins, interleukin-1 and interleukin-6 are also involved with regulating the immune system.

International Classification of Diseases and Related Health Problems— See ICD.

intestinal hyperpermeability (leaky gut)—An opening of the intestinal cell walls, or an opening up of the gut's mucosal barrier, which leads to chronic inflammation and thus to chronic disease. The breakdown of the gut barrier lets bacteria and toxins into the body's circulation, causing the immune system to work overtime.

J–K

Kallmann's syndrome—Form of hypogonadism caused by congenital gonadotropin-releasing hormone (GnRH) deficiency. It is a condition that lacks the pituitary hormones LH and FSH, and thus presents the body with delayed puberty. It is more common in males, with many of them not having the sense of smell.

Klinefelter's syndrome—Most common congenital abnormality in males causing primary hypogonadism (testicular failure). Occurring in approximately one in 1,000 live male births, this syndrome is the clinical manifestation of a male who has an extra X chromosome.

L

leaky gut—See intestinal hyperpermeability.

LH (luteinizing hormone)—Necessary for proper reproductive function. In women it triggers ovulation, while in men it is involved in testosterone production.

longevity gene (Sirtuin 1 gene)—Activation of the Sirtuin 1 gene is believed to increase longevity. Resveratrol (supplement) has been shown to activate the Sirtuin 1 gene, which is the same gene that is activated with a very low calorie diet—but without the hunger.

low blood sugar—See hypoglycemia.

luteinizing hormone—See LH.

M

melatonin—Hormone that is produced in the pineal gland (in the brain) and helps with the sleep cycle. Melatonin is also an important antioxidant, and is involved with the immune system.

menopause—When the ovaries stop making estrogen and the monthly (menstrual) periods stop. Surgical menopause happens when the ovaries are surgically removed while a woman is still having menstrual cycles. Menopause is the dramatic decline in estrogen that impacts many organs including brain, skin, bone and heart.

metabolism—the complete set of chemical reactions inside a cell. The metabolism of an organism determines what it finds nutritious, the pace at which it converts nutrients to energy, and how it stores excess nutrients.

metabolic syndrome—Metabolic risk factors that increase the chances of developing heart disease, stroke, and diabetes. Genetic factors, too much body fat, eating too many refined sugars, having prediabetes, having high blood pressure, having a high triglyceride level, and a lack of exercise all add to the development of this condition. It is a reversible condition with proper diet, exercise, life style modification and taking proper supplements.

mild thyroid failure (subclinical hypothyroidism)—Condition in which the thyroid is considered to be slowly failing. Blood tests will indicate mild thyroid failure when the TSH (thyroid stimulating hormone) is above three; however, in conventional medicine, it will not be considered until the TSH reaches five or higher. A normal TSH should be around one. Symptoms may include tiredness, cold intolerance, constipation, dry skin, depression, low libido, brittle fingernails and weight gain.

N

necrosis—Death of a cell either from infection, toxin or trauma.

nuclear factor kappa beta (NFKB)—A protein complex that plays a key role in stress. NFKB controls the reading of the DNA, and are considered first responders to a toxic event like an infection. Once activated it can turn on the DNA to make other chemicals to respond to the toxic event. Incorrect regulation of NFKB has been linked to cancer, a weak immune system and autoimmune diseases.

O

obesity—Typically defined with a body mass Index (BMI) above 30. A BMI is derived from the weight and height of a person. Obesity increases mortality and the likelihood in developing heart disease, diabetes, cancer and sleep apnea. A BMI of 30 or more will usually reveal obesity; although, weight lifters with more muscle and lower amounts of body fat may also have a BMI over 30. Therefore, the best test is to measure the amount of body fat that a person has. Generally, a body fat of 30 percent or more is considered obese.

omega-3—Fatty acids that have been shown to reduce inflammation and may help prevent chronic diseases, such as heart disease and arthritis. In the body, these essential fatty acids are highly concentrated in the brain and may be particularly important for cognitive and behavioral health as well as normal growth and development. Important omega-3 fatty acids include ALA (alpha-linolenic acid), EPA (eicosapentaenoic acid) and DHA (docosahexaenoic acid).

orchitis—Painful inflammation of the testicles that can lead to hypo-gonadism.

osteoporosis—The diminishing of bone density, typically related to ag-ing, low vitamin D levels and menopause in women. Also, osteopo-rosis happens in men with low testosterone and low vitamin D lev-els. Other causes are steroid induced bone loss, overactive thyroid and also hyperparathyroidism (high levels of parathyroid hormones that cause calcium to be lost from the bones).

ovaries—The egg producing organs found in females, they produce the hormones estrogen and progesterone

oxytocin—Hormone that acts as a neurotransmitter in the brain, facili-tating birth and breastfeeding. Has also been shown to play a role in the achievement of orgasm.

P

pangamic acid—See dimethylglycine.

pancreas—Organ that helps with digestion and also secretes several hormones including amylin, somatostatin, glucagon and insulin. Insulin is a hormone that helps glucose move from the blood into the cells where it is used for energy. The pancreas also secretes glucagon when the blood sugar is low to raise the glucose levels. Amylin is a hormone that is co-secreted with insulin to help lower glucose differ-ently from insulin. Somatostatin regulates the secretion of insulin and glucagon.

parathyroid—Located behind the thyroid gland are four tiny parathyroid glands which make hormones that help control calcium and phosphorous levels in the body. The parathyroid glands are necessary for proper bone development.

PC (phosphatidylcholine)—Fat, or lipid, in the cell membranes of the body's 100 trillion cells. Also found in proteins. PC is the main source of a neurotransmitter of acetylcholine.

perimenopause—Condition just before menopause, which may occur ten years before menopause begins. Symptoms of perimenopause are night sweats, hot flashes, irregular periods, mood changes, vaginal dryness and loss of libido.

phosphatidylcholine—See PC.

pineal gland—Small endocrine gland located in the center of the brain between the two hemispheres. It secretes melatonin, which helps regulate wake/sleep patterns.

pituitary gland—Small endocrine gland located at the base of the skull, this pea-sized gland helps control growth, blood pressure, breast milk production and metabolism. The pituitary gland plays an important role in growth, fluid balance, thyroid function and puberty, just to name a few.

PMS (premenstrual syndrome)—The appearance of physical and emotional symptoms during the second half of the menstrual cycle. Usual symptoms happen about 1 to 2 weeks before the period with issues of emotional instability, shorter fuse, water retention, insomnia, headaches and constipation.

polycystic ovary syndrome (PCOS)—An endocrine disorder with a host of symptoms related to small painful cysts on the ovaries. It is marked by the overproduction of male hormones in females. PCOS presents itself with irregular periods, is a leading cause of infertility and is related with metabolic syndrome or with insulin resistance.

Prader-Willi syndrome—Genetic disorder that can cause a growth hormone deficiency. It is marked by small stature, learning difficulties and a preoccupation with food.

premenstrual syndrome—See PMS.

progesterone—Female hormone that acts on the uterus (womb) to prepare it for receiving an egg following fertilization. When progesterone levels go down each month, this causes the bleeding associated with menstrual (monthly) periods. Progesterone is a hormone that can help prevent breast cancer and prostate cancer, helps with insomnia, improves bones and also helps with reducing anxiety. Progesterone is also produced in men but in much smaller quantities.

progestin—Synthetic form of progesterone, this class of drugs was developed in the 1950s to allow absorption by mouth for use in birth control pills. Medroxyprogesterone is also considered progestin, or synthetic progesterone, and not bioidentical progesterone. Provera® has medroxyprogesterone acetate.

prolactin—Hormone that helps with breast milk production. High levels of estrogen during pregnancy stimulate its production. Prolactin is made in the pituitary gland.

Q

quinones—Organic compounds that are found naturally in the environment and in our bodies; however, quinones can rapidly form into free radicals that cause oxidative damage to cells. Quinone reductase is an important enzyme in neutralizing quinones.

R

resveratrol—Chemical that is found in the skin of red grapes and in red wine that may have an effect of improving longevity. In animal studies, resveratrol has been shown to be anti-inflammatory and have anti-cancer effects. Resveratrol has also been shown to activate the Sirtuin 1 gene that is believed to be involved with longevity. Drinking one glass of red wine has about one milligram of resveratrol, whereas I recommend a dose over 200 mg. Resveratrol comes in a pill form.

S

sex hormone binding globulin (SHBG)—Carrier protein that binds to the hormones testosterone and estradiol. SHBG is mostly produced in the liver. Conditions with low levels of SHBG include polycystic ovary syndrome, diabetes and hypothyroidism. Conditions with high SHBG include pregnancy, hyperthyroidism, and anorexia nervosa.

SHBG—See sex hormone binding globulin.

Sirtuin 1 gene—See longevity gene.

sleep apnea—Condition where one stops breathing while sleeping. Significant levels are when one stops breathing more than five times per hour. An overnight sleep study is needed to make a proper diagnosis.

steroid—Any of various molecules, including hormones, that contain a particular arrangement of carbon rings. Some common steroids include sex steroids, corticosteroids, anabolic steroids and cholesterol.

subclinical hypothyroidism—See mild thyroid failure.

sublingual delivery (under the tongue delivery)—Method of delivering medications under the tongue, which bypasses the liver. Sublingual is considered a transmucosal route of delivery.

T

T cells—A certain type of white blood cells that are involved with the immune system. Certain T cells assist other white blood cells and are called T helper cells. Another class of T cells, cytotoxic T cells, destroy virally infected cells and tumor cells.

testes—Male reproductive organs, they produce sperm and the hormone testosterone.

testosterone—As a steroid, an androgen hormone and the primary male sex hormone, testosterone is produced by the testes in men and ovaries in women. It plays key roles in libido, energy and the immune function in both men and women. Testosterone also helps with muscle and bone formation, and also with hair growth.

thymus—Gland located in the chest just behind the sternum. Hormones produced by this gland stimulate the production of certain infection-fighting cells, and play a central role in the development of T cells.

thyroid—Gland located inside the neck, it regulates metabolism, which is the body's ability to break down food and convert it to energy. The thyroid gland secretes the hormones thyroxine (T4), triiodothyronine (T3), and calcitonin. The thyroid also is involved in growth. Thyroid disorders result from too little or too much thyroid hormone. Symptoms of hypothyroidism (too little hormone) include decreased energy, slow heart rate, dry skin, constipation, irritability, increased serum cholesterol, irregular menstrual cycles and feeling cold.

thyroid-stimulating hormone (TSH or thyrotropin)—Stimulates the thyroid to secrete the hormones thyroxine (T4) and triiodothyronine

(T3). TSH is made in the anterior pituitary gland and regulates the thyroid to make more or less of the thyroid hormones, T4 and T3.

thyrotropin-releasing hormone (TRH)—A hormone produced in the hypothalamus that regulates TSH.

thyrotropin—See thyroid-stimulating hormone.

TNF (tumor necrosis factor)—A class of chemical substances involved with inflammation, that is used to measure inflammation. TNF is considered a cytokine (chemical substance) that is involved with cell death. Too much production of TNF has been linked to cancer and chronic health disease (e.g., rheumatoid arthritis).

total testosterone—Total amount of testosterone in the blood, combining free testosterone and testosterone bound to certain molecules and already at use in the body (SHBG).

transdermal delivery—Method of delivering medications through the skin, it may be accomplished through patches that are worn for varying lengths of time, or as an ointment that is applied manually.

TRH—See thyrotropin-releasing hormone.

TSH—See thyroid-stimulating hormone.

tumor necrosis factor—See TNF.

Turner syndrome—occurs in females when one of the X (female) chromosomes is missing or damaged. The most common features are short stature and reduced or absent development of the ovaries. As adults, women with this disorder are typically infertile.

U

under the tongue delivery—See sublingual delivery.

V

vitamin D—A fat soluble vitamin that can be found in some foods, but is mostly made by the skin when exposed to ultraviolet rays from the sun. Active vitamin D functions as a hormone because it sends messages to the intestines to increase the absorption of calcium and phosphorus. Vitamin D deficiency is known to cause several bone diseases, including rickets and osteoporosis. Improving on vitamin D levels can reduce the risk of certain cancers and improve the immune system. Vo2 Max

Vo2 Max—Sophisticated testing equipment used by the National Olympic Training Center (and by Duke University, University of Florida and John Hopkins) to accurately determine individual levels of cardiovascular fitness.

W—Z

xenoestrogens—Man-made chemicals that have an estrogen effect. The concern about xenoestrogens is that they act as false messengers that disrupt the reproduction system. Some chemicals that have estrogen effects are DDT (insecticide), bisphenol A (found in plastics) and phthalates (plasticizers).

References

Chapter 1: Leaky Gut

[1] Fukui, A., et al. "Acetyl salicylic acid induces damage to intestinal epithelial cells by oxidation-related modifications of ZO-1." Am J Physiol Gastrointest Liver Physiol, 2012 Oct 15;303(8):G927-36.

[2] Lambert, G.P., et al. "Effect of aspirin dose on gastrointestinal permeability." Int J Sports Med, 2012 Jun;33(6):421-5.

[3] Lebedeva, V.V., et al. "[Hyperpermeability of the small intestine mucosa after prolonged application of non-steroidal anti-inflammatory drugs in patients with rheumatic diseases]." [Article in Russian] Eksp Klin Gastroenterol, 2008;(2):16-21.

[4] Tachecí, I., et al. "Non-steroidal anti-inflammatory drug induced injury to the small intestine." Acta Medica (Hradec Kralove), 2010;53(1):3-11.

[5] Ventura, M.T., et al. "Intestinal permeability in patients with adverse reactions to food." Dig Liver Dis, 2006 Oct;38(10):732-6.

[6] Perrier. C. and Corthésy, B. "Gut permeability and food allergies." Clin Exp Allergy, 2011 Jan;41(1):20-8.

[7] Yu, L.C. "The epithelial gatekeeper against food allergy." Pediatr Neonatol, 2009 Dec;50(6):247-54.

8 van Ampting, M.T., et al. "Damage to the intestinal epithelial barrier by antibiotic pretreatment of salmonella-infected rats is lessened by dietary calcium or tannic acid." J Nutr, 2010 Dec;140(12):2167-72.

9 Wood, S., et al. "Chronic alcohol exposure renders epithelial cells vulnerable to bacterial infection." PLoS One, 2013;8(1):e54646.

10 Chang, B., et al. "The role of FoxO4 in the relationship between alcohol-induced intestinal barrier dysfunction and liver injury." Int J Mol Med, 2013 Mar;31(3):569-76.

11 Wardill, H.R., et al. "Chemotherapy-induced gut toxicity: are alterations to intestinal tight junctions pivotal?" Cancer Chemother Pharmacol, 2012 Nov;70(5):627-35.

12 Melichar, B. and Zezulová, M. "The significance of altered gastrointestinal permeability in cancer patients." Curr Opin Support Palliat Care, 2011 Mar;5(1):47-54.

13 Fasano, A. "Intestinal permeability and its regulation by zonulin: diagnostic and therapeutic implications." Clin Gastroenterol Hepatol, 2012 Oct;10(10):1096-100.

14 Duerksen, D.R., et al. "A comparison of antibody testing, permeability testing, and zonulin levels with small-bowel biopsy in celiac disease patients on a gluten-free diet." Dig Dis Sci, 2010 Apr;55(4):1026-31.

15 Vighi, G. "Allergy and the gastrointestinal system." Clin Exp Immunol, 21 Juj 2008 DOI: 10.1111/j.1365-2249.2008.03713.x

16 Fasano, A. "Leaky gut and autoimmune diseases." Clin Rev Allergy Immunol, 2012 Feb;42(1):71-8.

17 Vaarala, O. "The "perfect storm" for type 1 diabetes: the complex interplay between intestinal microbiota, gut permeability, and mucosal immunity." Diabetes, 2008 Oct;57(10):2555-62.

18 Watts, T. "Role of the intestinal tight junction modulator zonulin in the pathogenesis of type I diabetes in BB diabetic-prone rats." Proc Natl Acad Sci U S A, 2005 Feb 22;102(8):2916-21.

19 Moreno-Navarrete, J.M., et al. "Circulating zonulin, a marker of intestinal permeability, is increased in association with obesity-associated insulin resistance." PLoS One, 2012;7(5):e37160.

20 Fasano, A. "Leaky gut and autoimmune diseases." Clin Rev Allergy Immunol, 2012 Feb;42(1):71-8.

21 Duerksen, D.R., et al. "A comparison of antibody testing, permeability testing, and zonulin levels with small-bowel biopsy in celiac disease patients on a gluten-free diet." Dig Dis Sci, 2010 Apr;55(4):1026-31.

22 Visser, J., et al. "Tight junctions, intestinal permeability, and auto-immunity: celiac disease and type 1 diabetes paradigms." Ann N Y Acad Sci, 2009 May;1165:195-205.

23 Yacyshyn, B., et al. "Multiple sclerosis patients have peripheral blood CD45RO+ B cells and increased intestinal permeability." Dig Dis Sci, 1996 Dec;41(12):2493-8.

24 Fasano, A. "Zonulin and its regulation of intestinal barrier function: the biological door to inflammation, autoimmunity, and cancer." Physiol Rev, 2011 Jan;91(1):151-75.

25 Pham, M., et al. "Subclinical intestinal inflammation in siblings of children with Crohn's disease." Dig Dis Sci, 2010 Dec;55(12):3502-7.

26 D'Incà, R., et al. "Increased intestinal permeability and NOD2 variants in familial and sporadic Crohn's disease." Aliment Pharmacol Ther, 2006 May 15;23(10):1455-61.

27 Irvine, E.J. and Marshall, J.K. "Increased intestinal permeability precedes the onset of Crohn's disease in a subject with familial risk." Gastroenterology, 2000 Dec;119(6):1740-4.

28 Weber, C.R. and Turner, J.R. "Inflammatory bowel disease: is it really just another break in the wall?" Gut, 2007;56:6-8

29 Lin, J.E., et al. "GUCY2C opposes systemic genotoxic tumorigenesis by regulating AKT-dependent intestinal barrier integrity." PLoS One, 2012;7(2):e31686.

30 Fasano, A. "Zonulin and its regulation of intestinal barrier function: the biological door to inflammation, autoimmunity, and cancer." Physiol Rev, 2011 Jan;91(1):151-75.

31 Kang, S.M., et al. "The Haptoglobin β chain as a supportive biomarker for human lung cancers." Mol Biosyst, 2011 Apr;7(4):1167-75.

32 Tsai, H.Y., et al. "Glycoproteomics analysis to identify a glycoform on haptoglobin associated with lung cancer." Proteomics, 2011 Jun;11(11):2162-70.

33 Arnold, J.N., et al. "Novel glycan biomarkers for the detection of lung cancer." J Proteome Res, 2011 Apr 1;10(4):1755-64.

34 Mandato, V.D., et al. "Haptoglobin phenotype and epithelial ovarian cancer." Anticancer Res, 2012 Oct;32(10):4353-8.

35 Tabassum, U., et al. "Elevated serum haptoglobin is associated with clinical outcome in triple-negative breast cancer patients." Asian Pac J Cancer Prev, 2012;13(9):4541-4.

36 Mishra, A. and Makharia, G.K. "Techniques of functional and motility test: how to perform and interpret intestinal permeability." J Neurogastroenterol Motil, 2012 Oct;18(4):443-7.

37 Fasano, A. "Zonulin and its regulation of intestinal barrier function: the biological door to inflammation, autoimmunity, and cancer." Physiol Rev, 2011 Jan;91(1):151-75.

38 Ortolani, C., et al. "Food allergies and food intolerances." Best Pract Res Clin Gastroenterol, 2006;20(3):467-83.

39 Tarlo, S.M. and Sussman, G.L. "Asthma and anaphylactoid reactions to food additives." Minerva Pediatr, 2008 Dec;60(6):1401-9.

40 MacDermott, R.P. "Treatment of irritable bowel syndrome in outpatients with inflammatory bowel disease using a food and beverage intolerance, food and beverage avoidance diet." Inflamm Bowel Dis, 2007 Jan;13(1):91-6.

41 Maintz, L. and Novak, N. "Histamine and histamine intolerance." Am J Clin Nutr, 2007 May;85(5):1185-96.

42 Lang, C.A., et al. "Symptom prevalence and clustering of symptoms in people living with chronic hepatitis C infection." J Pain Symptom Manage, 2006 Apr;31(4):335-44.

43 Liu, Z.H., et al. "The effects of perioperative probiotic treatment on serum zonulin concentration and subsequent postoperative infectious complications after colorectal cancer surgery: a double-center and double-blind randomized clinical trial." Am J Clin Nutr, 2013 Jan;97(1):117-26.

44 Lamprecht, M., et al. "Probiotic supplementation affects markers of intestinal barrier, oxidation, and inflammation in trained men; a randomized, double-blinded, placebo-controlled trial." J Int Soc Sports Nutr, 2012 Sep 20;9(1):45.

45 Ukena, S.N., et al. "Probiotic Escherichia coli Nissle 1917 inhibits leaky gut by enhancing mucosal integrity." PLoS One, 2007 Dec 12;2(12):e1308.

46 Rapin, J.R. and Wiernsperger, N. "Possible links between intestinal permeability and food processing: A potential therapeutic niche for glutamine." Clinics (Sao Paulo), 2010 Jun;65(6):635-43.

47 Everard, A., et al. "Tetrahydro iso-alpha acids from hops improve glucose homeostasis and reduce body weight gain and metabolic endotoxemia in high-fat diet-fed mice." PLoS One, 2012;7(3):e33858.

Chapter 2: Adrenal Fatigue

[1] Raison, C.L., et al. "Interferon-alpha effects on diurnal hypothalamic-pituitary-adrenal axis activity: relationship with proinflammatory cytokines and behavior." Mol Psychiatry, 2010 May;15(5):535-47.

[2] Bunevicius, A., et al. "Fatigue in patients with coronary artery disease: association with thyroid axis hormones and cortisol." Psychosom Med, 2012 Oct;74(8):848-53.

[3] Papadopoulos, A.S. and Cleare, A.J. "Hypothalamic-pituitary-adrenal axis dysfunction in chronic fatigue syndrome." Nat Rev Endocrinol, 2011 Sep 27;8(1):22-32.

[4] Urhausen, A., et al. "Impaired pituitary hormonal response to exhaustive exercise in overtrained endurance athletes." Med Sci Sports Exerc, 1998 Mar;30(3):407-14.

[5] Wetsch, W.A., et al. "Preoperative stress and anxiety in day-care patients and inpatients undergoing fast-track surgery." Br J Anaesth, 2009 Aug;103(2):199-205.

[6] Vreeburg, S.A., et al. "Major depressive disorder and hypothalamic-pituitary-adrenal axis activity: results from a large cohort study." Arch Gen Psychiatry, 2009 Jun;66(6):617-26.

[7] Jäger, R., et al. "Phospholipids and sports performance." J Int Soc Sports Nutr, 2007 Jul 25;4:5.

[8] Hellhammer, J., et al. "Effects of soy lecithin phosphatidic acid and phosphatidylserine complex (PAS) on the endocrine and psychological responses to mental stress." Stress, 2004 Jun;7(2):119-26.

Chapter 3: Hypothyroidism

[1] Wartofsky, L. and Dickey, R.A. "The evidence for a narrower thyrotropin reference range is compelling." J Clin Endocrinol Metab, 2005 Sep;90(9):5483-8.

2 Felig, P. and Frohman, L.A. Endocrinology and Metabolism. New York: McGraw-Hill, 2001. Print.

3 Bunevicius, R., et al. "Effects of thyroxine as compared with thyroxine plus triiodothyronine in patients with hypothyroidism." N Engl J Med, 1999 Feb 11;340(6):424-9.

4 Clyde, P.W., et al. "Combined levothyroxine plus liothyronine compared with levothyroxine alone in primary hypothyroidism: a randomized controlled trial." JAMA, 2003 Dec 10;290(22):2952-8.

5 Escobar-Morreale, H.F., et al. "Treatment of hypothyroidism with combinations of levothyroxine plus liothyronine." J Clin Endocrinol Metab, 2005 Aug;90(8):4946-54.

6 Escobar-Morreale, H.F., et al. "Thyroid hormone replacement therapy in primary hypothyroidism: a randomized trial comparing L-thyroxine plus liothyronine with L-thyroxine alone." Ann Intern Med, 2005 Mar 15;142(6):412-24.

7 Joffe, R.T., et al. "Treatment of clinical hypothyroidism with thyroxine and triiodothyronine: a literature review and meta-analysis." Psychosomatics, 2007 Sep-Oct;48(5):379-84.

8 Danzi, S. and Klein, I. "Thyroid hormone and the cardiovascular system." Minerva Endocrinol, 2004 Sep;29(3):139-50.

9 Kokkonen, L, et al. "Atrial fibrillation in elderly patients after cardiac surgery: postoperative hemodynamics and low postoperative serum triiodothyronine." J Cardiothorac Vasc Anesth, 2005 Apr;19(2):182-7.

10 Iervasi, G., et al. "Low-T3 syndrome: a strong prognostic predictor of death in patients with heart disease." Circulation, 2003 Feb 11;107(5):708-13.

11 Pingitore, A., et al. "Acute effects of triiodothyronine (T3) replacement therapy in patients with chronic heart failure and low-T3 syndrome: a randomized, placebo-controlled study." J Clin Endocrinol Metab, 2008 Apr;93(4):1351-8, Epub 2008 Jan 2.

[12] Park, Y.J., et al. "Subclinical hypothyroidism might increase the risk of transient atrial fibrillation after coronary artery bypass grafting." Ann Thorac Surg, 2009 Jun;87(6):1846-52.

[13] Asvold, B.O., et al. "Association between blood pressure and serum thyroid-stimulating hormone concentration within the reference range: a population-based study." J Clin Endocrinol Metab, 2007 Mar;92(3):841-5.

[14] Roos, A., et al. "Thyroid function is associated with components of the metabolic syndrome in euthyroid subjects." J Clin Endocrinol Metab, 2007 Feb;92(2):491-6.

[15] Quan, M.L., et al. "Bone mineral density in well-differentiated thyroid cancer patients treated with suppressive thyroxine: a systematic overview of the literature." J Surg Oncol, 2002 Jan;79(1):62-9; discussion 69-70.

[16] Görres, G., et al. "Bone mineral density in patients receiving suppressive doses of thyroxine for differentiated thyroid carcinoma." Eur J Nucl Med, 1996 Jun;23(6):690-2.

[17] Quan, M.L., et al. "Bone mineral density in well-differentiated thyroid cancer patients treated with suppressive thyroxine: a systematic overview of the literature." J Surg Oncol, 2002 Jan;79(1):62-9; discussion 69-70.

[18] Bianco, A.C., et al. "Biochemistry, cellular and molecular biology, and physiological roles of the iodothyronine selenodeiodinases." Endocr Rev, 2002 Feb;23(1):38-89.

[19] Bianco, A.C., et al. "Biochemistry, cellular and molecular biology, and physiological roles of the iodothyronine selenodeiodinases." Endocr Rev, 2002 Feb;23(1):38-89.

[20] Green, J.R. "Thyroid function in chronic liver disease." Z Gastroenterol, 1979 Jul;17(7):447-51.

[21] Panicker, V. et al. "Common variation in the DIO2 gene predicts baseline psychological well-being and response to combination thy-

roxine plus triiodothyronine therapy in hypothyroid patients." J Clin
Endocrinol Metab, 2009 May;94(5):1623-9.

[22] Butler, P.W., et al. "The Thr92Ala 5' type 2 deiodinase gene polymorphism is associated with a delayed triiodothyronine secretion in
response to the thyrotropin-releasing hormone-stimulation test: a
pharmacogenomic study." Thyroid, 2010 Dec;20(12):1407-12.

[23] Al-Azzam, S.I., et al. "The Role of Type II Deiodinase Polymorphisms in Clinical Management of Hypothyroid Patients Treated
with Levothyroxine." Exp Clin Endocrinol Diabetes, 2013 Jan 17.

[24] Wiersinga, W.M. "Do we need still more trials on T4 and T3 combination therapy in hypothyroidism?" Eur J Endocrinol, 2009
Dec;161(6):955-9.

Chapter 4: Estrogen

[1] Rossouw, J.E., et al. "Risks and benefits of estrogen plus progestin in
healthy postmenopausal women: principal results from the Women's
Health Initiative randomized controlled trial." JAMA, 2002 Jul
17;288(3):321-33.

[2] Randal, J. "The end of an era? Study reveals harms of hormone replacement therapy." J Natl Cancer Inst, 2002 Aug 7;94(15):1116-8.

[3] de Lignières, B., et al. "Combined hormone replacement therapy and
risk of breast cancer in a French cohort study of 3175 women." Climacteric, 2002 Dec;5(4):332-40.

[4] Dunn, L.B., et al. "Does estrogen prevent skin aging? Results from
the First National Health and Nutrition Examination Survey
(NHANES I)." Arch Dermatol, 1997 Mar;133(3):339-42.

[5] Schmidt, J.B., et al. "Treatment of skin aging with topical estrogens."
Int J Dermatol, 1996 Sep;35(9):669-74.

[6] Wolff, E.F., et al. "Long-term effects of hormone therapy on skin ri-
gidity and wrinkles." Fertil Steril, 2005 Aug;84(2):285-8.

7 Friday, K., et al. "Conjugated Equine Estrogen Improves Glycemic Control and Blood Lipoproteins in Postmenopausal Women with Type 2 Diabetes." J Clin Endocrinol Metab, 2001 Jan;86(1):48-52.

8 Huffman, K.M., et al. "Impact of hormone replacement therapy on exercise training-induced improvements in insulin action in sedentary overweight adults." Metabolism, 2008 Jul;57(7):888-95.

9 Simpkins, J.W., et al. "Role of estrogen replacement therapy in memory enhancement and the prevention of neuronal loss associated with Alzheimer's disease." Am J Med, 1997 Sep 22;103(3A):19S-25S.

10 Greene, R.A. and Dixon, W. "The role of reproductive hormones in maintaining cognition." Obstet Gynecol Clin North Am, 2002 Sep;29(3):437-53.

11 Cauley, J.A., et al. "Timing of estrogen replacement therapy for optimal osteoporosis prevention." J Clin Endocrinol Metab, 2001 Dec;86(12):5700-5.

12 Harman, S.M. "Estrogen replacement in menopausal women: recent and current prospective studies, the WHI and the KEEPS." Gend Med, 2006 Dec;3(4):254-69.

13 Mosca, L., et al. "Evidence-based guidelines for cardiovascular disease prevention in women: 2007 update." Circulation, 2007 Mar 20;115(11):1481-501.

14 Friday, K., et al. "Conjugated Equine Estrogen Improves Glycemic Control and Blood Lipoproteins in Postmenopausal Women with Type 2 Diabetes." J Clin Endocrinol Metab, 2001 Jan;86(1):48-52.

15 Huffman, K.M., et al. "Impact of hormone replacement therapy on exercise training-induced improvements in insulin action in sedentary overweight adults." Metabolism, 2008 Jul;57(7):888-95.

16 Shifren, J.L., et al. "A comparison of the short-term effects of oral conjugated equine estrogens versus transdermal estradiol on C-reactive protein, other serum markers of inflammation, and other

hepatic proteins in naturally menopausal women." J Clin Endocrinol Metab, 2008 May;93(5):1702-10.

[17] Lakoski, S.G. and Herrington, D.M. "Effects of hormone therapy on C-reactive protein and IL-6 in postmenopausal women: a review article." Climacteric, 2005 Dec;8(4):317-26.

[18] Canonico, M. and Scarabin, P.Y. "Hormone therapy and risk of venous thromboembolism among postmenopausal women." Climacteric, 2009;12 Suppl 1:76-80.

[19] L'hermite, M., et al. "Could transdermal estradiol + progesterone be a safer postmenopausal HRT? A review." Maturitas, 2008 Jul-Aug;60(3-4):185-201.

[20] van der Klaauw, A.A., et al. "Administration route-dependent effects of estrogens on IGF-I levels during fixed GH replacement in women with hypopituitarism." Eur J Endocrinol, 2007 Dec;157(6):709-16.

[21] Sonnet, E., et al. "Effects of the route of oestrogen administration on IGF-1 and IGFBP-3 in healthy postmenopausal women: results from a randomized, placebo-controlled study." Clin Endocrinol (Oxf), 2007 May;66(5):626-31.

[22] Sanada, M., et al. "Substitution of transdermal estradiol during oral estrogen-progestin therapy in postmenopausal women: effects on hypertriglyceridemia." Menopause, 2004 May-Jun;11(3):331-6.

[23] Czarnecka, D., et al. "Influence of hormone replacement therapy on the quality of life in postmenopausal women with hypertension." Przegl Lek, 2000;57(7-8):397-401.

[24] Freedman, R.R. and Blacker, C.M. "Estrogen raises the sweating threshold in postmenopausal women with hot flashes." Fertil Steril, 2002 Mar;77(3):487-90.

[25] Hazzard, W.R. and Applebaum-Bowden, D. "Why women live longer than men: the biologic mechanism of the sex differential in longevity." Trans Am Clin Climatol Assoc, 1990;101:168-88.

[26] Joffe, H., et al. "Estrogen therapy selectively enhances prefrontal cognitive processes: a randomized, double-blind, placebo-controlled study with functional magnetic resonance imaging in perimenopausal and recently postmenopausal women." Menopause, 2006 May-Jun;13(3):411-22.

[27] Melamed, M., et al. "Molecular and kinetic basis for the mixed agonist/antagonist activity of estriol." Mol Endocrinol, 1997 Nov;11(12):1868-78.

[28] Scolozzi, R., et al. "Risk factors in breast cancer." Recenti Prog Med, 1981 May;70(5):463-86.

[29] Lagiou, P., et al. "Maternal height, pregnancy estriol and birth weight in reference to breast cancer risk in Boston and Shanghai." Int J Cancer, 2005 Nov 10;117(3):494-8.

[30] Bakken, K., et al. "Hormone replacement therapy and incidence of hormone-dependent cancers in the Norwegian Women and Cancer study." Int J Cancer, 2004 Oct 20;112(1):130-4.

[31] Hartman, J., et al. "Estrogen receptor beta in breast cancer—diagnostic and therapeutic implications." Steroids, 2009 Aug;74(8):635-41.

[32] Helguero, L.A., et al. "Estrogen receptors alfa (ERalpha) and beta (ERbeta) differentially regulate proliferation and apoptosis of the normal murine mammary epithelial cell line HC11." Oncogene, 2005 Oct 6;24(44):6605-16.

[33] Gustafsson, J.A. and Warner, M. "Estrogen receptor beta in the breast: role in estrogen responsiveness and development of breast cancer." J Steroid Biochem Mol Biol, 2000 Nov 30;74(5):245-8.

[34] Fox, E.M., et al. "ERbeta in breast cancer—onlooker, passive player, or active protector?" Steroids, 2008 Oct;73(11):1039-51.

[35] Sasano, H. and Harada, N. "Intratumoral aromatase in human breast, endometrial, and ovarian malignancies." Endocr Rev, 1998 Oct;19(5):593-607.

36 Harris, S.T., et al. "The effects of estrone (Ogen®) on spinal bone density of postmenopausal women." Arch Intern Med, 1991 Oct;151(10):1980-4.

37 Peck, J.D., et al. "Steroid hormone levels during pregnancy and incidence of maternal breast cancer." Cancer Epidemiol Biomarkers Prev, 2002 Apr;11(4):361-8.

38 Miettinen, M.M., et al.. "Human 17 beta-hydroxysteroid dehydrogenase type 1 and type 2 isoenzymes have opposite activities in cultured cells and characteristic cell—and tissue-specific expression." Biochem J, 1996 Mar 15;314 (Pt 3):839-45.

39 "SEER Stat Fact Sheets: Breast."
http://www.seer.cancer.gov/statfacts/html/breast.html

40 Foster, P.A. "Steroid metabolism in breast cancer." Minerva Endocrinol, 2008 Mar;33(1):27-37.

41 Poirier, D. "Advances in development of inhibitors of 17beta hydroxysteroid dehydrogenases." Anticancer Agents Med Chem, 2009 Jul;9(6):642-60.

42 Day, J.M., et al. "17beta-hydroxysteroid dehydrogenase Type 1, and not Type 12, is a target for endocrine therapy of hormone-dependent breast cancer." Int J Cancer, 2008 May 1;122(9):1931-40.

43 Deroo, B.J. and Korach, K.S. "Estrogen receptors and human disease." J Clin Invest, 2006 Mar;116(3):561-70.

44 Paruthiyil, S., et al. "Estrogen receptor beta inhibits human breast cancer cell proliferation and tumor formation by causing a G2 cell cycle arrest." Cancer Res, 2004 Jan 1;64(1):423-8.

45 Zhu, B.T., et al. "Quantitative structure-activity relationship of various endogenous estrogen metabolites for human estrogen receptor alpha and beta subtypes: Insights into the structural determinants favoring a differential subtype binding." Endocrinology, 2006 Sep;147(9):4132-50.

[46] Melamed, M., et al. "Molecular and kinetic basis for the mixed agonist/antagonist activity of estriol." Mol Endocrinol, 1997 Nov;11(12):1868-78.

[47] Baracat, E., et al. "Estrogen activity and novel tissue selectivity of delta8,9-dehydroestrone sulfate in postmenopausal women." J Clin Endocrinol Metab, 1999 Jun;84(6):2020-7.

[48] Isaksson, E., et al. "Expression of estrogen receptors (alpha, beta) and insulin-like growth factor-1 in breast tissue from surgically postmenopausal cynomolgus macaques after long-term treatment with HRT and tamoxifen." Breast, 2002 Aug;11(4):295-300.

[49] Pisha, E., et al. "Evidence that a metabolite of equine estrogens, 4-hydroxyequilenin, induces cellular transformation in vitro." Chem Res Toxicol, 2001 Jan;14(1):82-90.

[50] Shen, L., et al. "Alkylation of 2'-deoxynucleosides and DNA by the Premarin® metabolite 4-hydroxyequilenin semiquinone radical." Chem Res Toxicol, 1998 Feb;11(2):94-101.

[51] "Why Are There Still PMU Farms in Existence?" http://www.premarin.org

[52] Van Gorp, T. and Neven, P. "Endometrial safety of hormone replacement therapy: review of literature." Maturitas, 2002 Jun 25;42(2):93-104.

[53] Granberg, S., et al. "The effects of oral estriol on the endometrium in postmenopausal women." Maturitas, 2002 Jun 25;42(2):149-56.

[54] Weiderpass, E., et al. "Low-potency oestrogen and risk of endometrial cancer: a case-control study." Lancet, 1999 May 29;353(9167):1824-8.

[55] Vooijs, G.P. and Geurts, T.B. "Review of the endometrial safety during intravaginal treatment with estriol." Eur J Obstet Gynecol Reprod Biol, 1995 Sep;62(1):101-6.

56 Raz, R. and Stamm, W.E. "A controlled trial of intravaginal estriol in postmenopausal women with recurrent urinary tract infections." N Engl J Med, 1993 Sep 9;329(11):753-6.

57 Joyce, C. "Study: Gender-Bending Fish Widespread In U.S." http://www.npr.org/templates/story/story.php?storyId=112888785

58 Roy, J.R., et al. "Estrogen-like endocrine disrupting chemicals affecting puberty in humans--a review." Med Sci Monit, 2009 Jun;15(6):RA137-45.

59 Adlercreutz, H., et al. "Estrogen metabolism and excretion in Oriental and Caucasian women." J Natl Cancer Inst, 1994 Jul 20;86(14):1076-82.

60 Im, A., et al. "Urinary estrogen metabolites in women at high risk for breast cancer." Carcinogenesis, 2009 Sep;30(9):1532-5.

61 Kabat, G.C., et al. "Estrogen metabolism and breast cancer." Epidemiology, 2006 Jan;17(1):80-8.

62 Bolton, J.L. and Thatcher, G.R. "Potential mechanisms of estrogen quinone carcinogenesis." Chem Res Toxicol, 2008 Jan;21(1):93-101.

63 Fagerholm, R., et al. "NAD(P)H:quinone oxidoreductase 1 NQO1*2 genotype (P187S) is a strong prognostic and predictive factor in breast cancer." Nat Genet, 2008 Jul;40(7):844-53.

64 Lu, F., et al. "Resveratrol prevents estrogen-DNA adduct formation and neoplastic transformation in MCF-10F cells." Cancer Prev Res (Phila Pa), 2008 Jul;1(2):135-45.

65 Hsieh, T.C. and Wu, J.M. "Suppression of cell proliferation and gene expression by combinatorial synergy of EGCG, resveratrol and gamma-tocotrienol in estrogen receptor-positive MCF-7 breast cancer cells." Int J Oncol, 2008 Oct;33(4):851-9.

66 Elangovan, S. and Hsieh, T.C. "Control of cellular redox status and upregulation of quinone reductase NQO1 via Nrf2 activation by

alpha-lipoic acid in human leukemia HL-60 cells." Int J Oncol, 2008 Oct;33(4):833-8.

[67] Singh, S., et al. "Relative imbalances in the expression of estrogen-metabolizing enzymes in the breast tissue of women with breast carcinoma." Oncol Rep, 2005 Oct;14(4):1091-6.

[68] Cushman, M., et al. "Estrogen plus progestin and risk of venous thrombosis." JAMA, 2004 Oct 6;292(13):1573-80.

[69] Scarabin, P.Y., et al. "Effects of oral and transdermal estrogen/progesterone regimens on blood coagulation and fibrinolysis in postmenopausal women. A randomized controlled trial." Arterioscler Thromb Vasc Biol, 1997 Nov;17(11):3071-8.

[70] O'Sullivan, A.J., et al. "The route of estrogen replacement therapy confers divergent effects on substrate oxidation and body composition in postmenopausal women." J Clin Invest, 1998 Sep 1;102(5):1035-40.

[71] Simon, J.A. "What's new in hormone replacement therapy: focus on transdermal estradiol and micronized progesterone." Climacteric, 2012 Apr;15 Suppl 1:3-10.

[72] Murkes, D., et al. "Percutaneous estradiol/oral micronized progesterone has less-adverse effects and different gene regulations than oral conjugated equine estrogens/medroxyprogesterone acetate in the breasts of healthy women in vivo." Gynecol Endocrinol, 2012 Oct;28 Suppl 2:12-5.

[73] Sanders, J.L. and Newman, A.B. "Telomere Length in Epidemiology: A Biomarker of Aging, Age-Related Disease, Both, or Neither?" Epidemiol Rev, 2013 Jan 9. [Epub ahead of print]

[74] Mikhelson, V.M. and Gamaley, I.A. "Telomere shortening is a sole mechanism of aging in mammals." Curr Aging Sci, 2012 Dec 1;5(3):203-8.

75 Lee, D.C., et al. "Effect of long-term hormone therapy on telomere length in postmenopausal women." Yonsei Med J, 2005 Aug 31;46(4):471-9.

76 Bayne, S., et al. "Estrogen deficiency reversibly induces telomere shortening in mouse granulosa cells and ovarian aging in vivo." Protein Cell, 2011 Apr;2(4):333-46.

Chapter 5: Progesterone

1 Miller, H. "Response to 'The bioidentical hormone debate: are bioidentical hormones (estradiol, estriol, and progesterone) safer or more efficacious than commonly used synthetic versions in hormone replacement therapy?'" Postgrad Med, 2009 Jul;121(4):172.

2 Schumacher, M., et al. "Novel Perspectives for Progesterone in Hormone Replacement Therapy, with Special Reference to the Nervous System." Endocr Rev, 2007 Jun;28(4):387-439.

3 "The Endocrine Society® Position Statement on Bioidentical Hormones."
http://www.endo-society.org/advocacy/policy/upload/BH_positi on_Statement_final_10_25_06_w_Header.pdf

4 Holtorf, K. "The bioidentical hormone debate: are bioidentical hormones (estradiol, estriol, and progesterone) safer or more efficacious than commonly used synthetic versions in hormone replacement therapy?" Postgrad Med, 2009 Jan;121(1):73-85.

5 de Lignières, B. "Effects of progestogens on the postmenopausal breast." Climacteric, 2002 Sep;5(3):229-35.

6 Saitoh, M., et al. "Medroxyprogesterone acetate induces cell proliferation through up-regulation of cyclin D1 expression via phosphatidylinositol 3-kinase/Akt/nuclear factor-kappaB cascade in human breast cancer cells." Endocrinology, 2005 Nov;146(11):4917-25.

7 Formby, B. and Wiley, T.S. "Progesterone inhibits growth and induces apoptosis in breast cancer cells: inverse effects on Bcl-2 and p53." Ann Clin Lab Sci, 1998 Nov-Dec;28(6):360-9.

8 Chlebowski, R.T., et al. "Influence of Estrogen Plus Progestin on Breast Cancer and Mammography in Healthy Postmenopausal Women." JAMA, 2003 Jun 25;289(24):3243-53.

9 Colditz, G.A. and Rosner, B. "Cumulative risk of breast cancer to age 70 years according to risk factor status: data from the Nurses' Health Study." Am J Epidemiol, 2000 Nov 15;152(10):950-64.

10 Ross, R.K., et al. "Effect of hormone replacement therapy on breast cancer risk: estrogen versus estrogen plus progestin." J Natl Cancer Inst, 2000 Feb 16;92(4):328-32.

11 Ewertz, M., et al. "Hormone use for menopausal symptoms and risk of breast cancer. A Danish cohort study." Br J Cancer, 2005 Apr 11;92(7):1293-7.

12 Magnusson, C., et al. "Breast-cancer risk following long-term oestrogen—and oestrogen-progestin-replacement therapy." Int J Cancer, 1999 May 5;81(3):339-44.

13 Fournier, A., et al. "Unequal risks for breast cancer associated with different hormone replacement therapies: results from the E3N cohort study." Breast Cancer Res Treat, 2008 Jan;107(1):103-11.

14 Veronese, S.M. and Gambacorta, M. "Detection of Ki-67 proliferation rate in breast cancer. Correlation with clinical and pathologic features." Am J Clin Pathol, 1991 Jan;95(1):30-4.

15 Badwe, R.A., et al. "Serum progesterone at the time of surgery and survival in women with premenopausal operable breast cancer." Eur J Cancer, 1994;30A(4):445-8.

16 Mohr, P., et al. "Serum progesterone and prognosis in operable breast cancer." Br J Cancer, 1996 June;73(12):1552-5.

17 Micheli, A., et al. "Endogenous sex hormones and subsequent breast cancer in premenopausal women." Int J Cancer, 2004 Nov 1;112(2):312-8.

18 de Lignières, B., et al. "Combined hormone replacement therapy and risk of breast cancer in a French cohort study of 3175 women." Climacteric, 2002 Dec;5(4):332-40.

19 Chlebowski, R.T., et al. "Influence of Estrogen Plus Progestin on Breast Cancer and Mammography in Healthy Postmenopausal Women." JAMA, 2003 Jun 25;289(24):3243-53.

20 Canonico, M., et al. "Hormone therapy and venous thromboembolism among postmenopausal women: impact of the route of estrogen administration and progestogens: the ESTHER study." Circulation, 2007 Feb 20;115(7):840-5.

21 Rosano, G.M., et al. "Natural progesterone, but not medroxyprogesterone acetate, enhances the beneficial effect of estrogen on exercise-induced myocardial ischemia in postmenopausal women." J Am Coll Cardiol, 2000 Dec;36(7):2154-9.

22 Otsuki, M., et al. "Progesterone, but not medroxyprogesterone, inhibits vascular cell adhesion molecule-1 expression in human vascular endothelial cells." Arterioscler Thromb Vasc Biol, 2001 Feb;21(2):243-8.

23 The Writing Group for the PEPI Trial: Miller, V.T., et. al. "Effects of estrogen or estrogen/progestin regimens on heart disease risk factors in postmenopausal women. The Postmenopausal Estrogen/Progestin Interventions (PEPI) Trial." JAMA, 1995 Jan 18;273(3):199-208.

24 Mishra, R.G., et al. "Medroxyprogesterone acetate and dihydrotestosterone induce coronary hyperreactivity in intact male rhesus monkeys." J Clin Endocrinol Metab, 2005 Jun;90(6):3706-14.

[25] Morey, A.K., et al. "Estrogen and progesterone inhibit vascular smooth muscle proliferation." Endocrinology, 1997 Aug;138(8):3330-9.

[26] Houser, S.L., et al. "Serum lipids and arterial plaque load are altered independently with high-dose progesterone in hypercholesterolemic male rabbits." Cardiovasc Pathol, 2000 Nov-Dec;9(6):317-22.

[27] Adams, M.R., et al. "Medroxyprogesterone acetate antagonizes inhibitory effects of conjugated equine estrogens on coronary artery atherosclerosis." Arterioscler Thromb Vasc Biol, 1997 Jan;17(1):217-21.

[28] Otsuki, M., et al. "Progesterone, but not medroxyprogesterone, inhibits vascular cell adhesion molecule-1 expression in human vascular endothelial cells." Arterioscler Thromb Vasc Biol, 2001 Feb;21(2):243-8.

[29] Ma, J., et al. "Progesterone for acute traumatic brain injury." Cochrane Database Syst Rev, 2012 Oct 17; DOI:10.1002/14651858.CD008409.pub3.

[30] Aminmansour, B., et al. "Comparison of the administration of progesterone versus progesterone and vitamin D in improvement of outcomes in patients with traumatic brain injury: A randomized clinical trial with placebo group." Adv Biomed Res, 2012;1:58.

[31] Singh, M. and Su, C. "Progesterone and neuroprotection." Horm Behav, 2013 Feb;63(2):284-90.

[32] Shumaker, S.A., et al. "Estrogen plus progestin and the incidence of dementia and mild cognitive impairment in postmenopausal women: the Women's Health Initiative Memory Study: a randomized controlled trial." JAMA, 2003 May 28;289(20):2651-62.

[33] Sanders, J.L. and Newman, A.B. "Telomere Length in Epidemiology: A Biomarker of Aging, Age-Related Disease, Both, or Neither?" Epidemiol Rev, 2013 Jan 9. [Epub ahead of print]

34 Mikhelson, V.M. and Gamaley, I.A. "Telomere shortening is a sole mechanism of aging in mammals." Curr Aging Sci, 2012 Dec 1;5(3):203-8.

35 Lee, D.C., et al. "Effect of long-term hormone therapy on telomere length in postmenopausal women." Yonsei Med J, 2005 Aug 31;46(4):471-9.

Chapter 6: Testosterone

1 Travison, T.G., et al. "The relative contributions of aging, health, and lifestyle factors to serum testosterone decline in men." J Clin Endocrinol Metab, 2007 Feb;92(2):549-55.

2 Elmlinger, M.W., et al. "Reference intervals for testosterone, androstenedione and SHBG levels in healthy females and males from birth until old age." Clin Lab, 2005;51(11-12):625-32.

3 Maggio, M., et al. "The relationship between testosterone and molecular markers of inflammation in older men." J Endocrinol Invest, 2005;28(11 Suppl Proceedings):116-9.

4 Cornoldi, A., et al. "Effects of chronic testosterone administration on myocardial ischemia, lipid metabolism and insulin resistance in elderly male diabetic patients with coronary artery disease." Int J Cardiol, 2010 Jun 25;142(1):50-5.

5 Estcourt, S., et al. "The patient experience of services for thyroid eye disease in the United Kingdom: results of a nationwide survey." Eur J Endocrinol, 2009 Sep;161(3):483-7.

6 Shores, M.M., et al. "Testosterone Treatment and Mortality in Men with Low Testosterone Levels." J Clin Endocrinol Metab, 2012 Jun;97(6):2050-2058.

7 Kenny, A.M., et al. "Effects of transdermal testosterone on bone and muscle in older men with low bioavailable testosterone levels, low bone mass, and physical frailty." J Am Geriatr Soc, 2010 Jun;58(6):1134-43.

8 Jackson, G., et al. "Erectile dysfunction and coronary artery disease prediction: evidence-based guidance and consensus." Int J Clin Pract, 2010 Jun;64(7):848-57.

9 Gill, J.K., et al. "Androgens, growth factors, and risk of prostate cancer: the Multiethnic Cohort." Prostate, 2010 Jun 1;70(8):906-15.

10 Song, K., et al. "DHT Selectively Reverses Smad3-Mediated/TGF-{beta}-Induced Responses through Transcriptional Down-Regulation of Smad3 in Prostate Epithelial Cells." Mol Endocrinol, 2010 Oct;24(10):2019-29.

11 Parsons, J.K., et al. "Prospective study of serum dihydrotestosterone and subsequent risk of benign prostatic hyperplasia in community dwelling men: the Rancho Bernardo Study." J Urol, 2010 Sep;184(3):1040-4.

12 Ellem, S.J. and Risbridger, G.F. "Aromatase and regulating the estrogen:androgen ratio in the prostate gland." J Steroid Biochem Mol Biol, 2010 Feb 28;118(4-5):246-51.

13 Morgentaler, A. "Guilt by association: a historical perspective on Huggins, testosterone therapy, and prostate cancer." J Sex Med, 2008 Aug;5(8):1834-40.

14 Raynaud, J.P. "Testosterone deficiency syndrome: treatment and cancer risk." J Steroid Biochem Mol Biol, 2009 Mar;114(1-2):96-105.

15 Rinnab, L., et al. "Testosterone replacement therapy and prostate cancer. The current position 67 years after the Huggins myth." Urologe A, 2009 May;48(5):516-22.

16 Davis, S.R., et al. "Testosterone for low libido in postmenopausal women not taking estrogen." N Engl J Med, 2008 Nov 6;359(19):2005-17. doi: 10.1056/NEJMoa0707302.

17 Rariy, C.M., et al. "Higher serum free testosterone concentration in older women is associated with greater bone mineral density, lean body mass, and total fat mass: the cardiovascular health study." J Clin Endocrinol Metab, 2011 Apr;96(4):989-96.

18 Britto, R., et al. "Hormonal therapy with estradiol and testosterone implants: bone protection?" Gynecol Endocrinol, 2011 Feb;27(2):96-100.

19 Britto, R., et al. "Improvement of the lipid profile in post menopausal women who use estradiol and testosterone implants." Gynecol Endocrinol, 2012 Oct;28(10):767-9.

20 Davey, D.A. "Androgens in women before and after the menopause and post bilateral oophorectomy: clinical effects and indications for testosterone therapy." Womens Health (Lond Engl), 2012 Jul;8(4):437-46.

21 Hofling, M., et al. "Testosterone inhibits estrogen/progestogen-induced breast cell proliferation in postmenopausal women." Menopause, 2007 Mar-Apr;14(2):183-90.

22 Glaser, R. and Dimitrakakis, C. "Testosterone therapy in women: Myths and misconceptions." Maturitas, 2013 Feb 1. pii: S0378-5122(13)00012-1.

23 Stergiopoulos, K., et al. "Anabolic steroids, acute myocardial infarction and polycythemia: a case report and review of the literature." Vasc Health Risk Manag, 2008;4(6):1475-80.

24 Sanders, J.L. and Newman, A.B. "Telomere Length in Epidemiology: A Biomarker of Aging, Age-Related Disease, Both, or Neither?" Epidemiol Rev, 2013 Jan 9. [Epub ahead of print]

25 Mikhelson, V.M. and Gamaley, I.A. "Telomere shortening is a sole mechanism of aging in mammals." Curr Aging Sci, 2012 Dec 1;5(3):203-8.

26 Zhang, L., et al. "Testosterone therapy delays cardiomyocyte aging via an androgen receptor-independent pathway." Braz J Med Biol Res, 2011 Nov;44(11):1118-24.

Chapter 7: DHEA

1 Orentreich, N., et al. "Long-term longitudinal measurements of plasma dehydroepiandrosterone sulfate in normal men." J Clin Endocrinol Metab, 1992 Oct;75(4):1002-4.

2 Ahn, R.S., et al. "Salivary cortisol and DHEA levels in the Korean population: age-related differences, diurnal rhythm, and correlations with serum levels." Yonsei Med J, 2007 Jun 30;48(3):379-88.

3 "DHEA: Evidence for anti-aging claims is weak." http://www.mayoclinic.com/health/dhea/HA00084

4 Nawata, H., et al. "Adrenopause." Horm Res, 2004;62 Suppl 3:110-4.

5 Nair, K.S., et al. "DHEA in elderly women and DHEA or testosterone in elderly men." N Engl J Med, 2006 Oct 19;355(16):1647-59.

6 Morales, A.J., et al. "The effect of six months treatment with a 100 mg daily dose of dehydroepiandrosterone (DHEA) on circulating sex steroids, body composition and muscle strength in age-advanced men and women." Clin Endocrinol (Oxf), 1998 Oct;49(4):421-32.

7 Baulieu, E.E., et al. "Dehydroepiandrosterone (DHEA), DHEA sulfate, and aging: contribution of the DHEAge Study to a sociobiomedical issue." Proc Natl Acad Sci USA, 2000 Apr 11;97(8):4279-84.

8 Enomoto, M., et al. "Serum dehydroepiandrosterone sulfate levels predict longevity in men: 27-year follow-up study in a community-based cohort (Tanushimaru study)." J Am Geriatr Soc, 2008 Jun;56(6):994-8.

9 Arlt, W., et al. "Dehydroepiandrosterone replacement in women with adrenal insufficiency." N Engl J Med, 1999 Sep 30;341(14):1013-20.

10 Jankowski, C.M., et al. "Increases in bone mineral density in response to oral dehydroepiandrosterone replacement in older adults appear to be mediated by serum estrogens." J Clin Endocrinol Metab, 2008 Dec;93(12):4767-73.

11 Weiss, E.P., et al. "Dehydroepiandrosterone replacement therapy in older adults: 1- and 2-y effects on bone." Am J Clin Nutr, 2009 May;89(5):1459-67.

12 Morales, A.J., et al. "Effects of replacement dose of dehydroepiandrosterone in men and women of advancing age." J Clin Endocrinol Metab, 1994 Jun;78(6):1360-7.

13 Straub, R.H., et al. "Association of humoral markers of inflammation and dehydroepiandrosterone sulfate or cortisol serum levels in patients with chronic inflammatory bowel disease." Am J Gastroenterol, 1998 Nov;93(11):2197-202.

14 Straub, R.H., et al. "Inadequately low serum levels of steroid hormones in relation to interleukin-6 and tumor necrosis factor in untreated patients with early rheumatoid arthritis and reactive arthritis." Arthritis Rheum, 2002 Mar;46(3):654-62.

15 Suzuki, N., et al. "Hormones and lupus: defective dehydroepiandrosterone activity induces impaired interleukin-2 activity of T lymphocytes in patients with systemic lupus erythematosus." Ann Med Interne (Paris), 1996;147(4):248-52.

16 Nordmark, G., et al. "Effects of dehydroepiandrosterone supplement on health-related quality of life in glucocorticoid treated female patients with systemic lupus erythematosus." Autoimmunity, 2005 Nov;38(7):531-40.

17 Straub, R.H., et al. "Replacement therapy with DHEA plus corticosteroids in patients with chronic inflammatory diseases — substitutes

of adrenal and sex hormones." Z Rheumatol, 2000;59 Suppl 2:II/108-18.

[18] Yang, S.C., et al. "Interactive effect of an acute bout of resistance exercise and dehydroepiandrosterone administration on glucose tolerance and serum lipids in middle-aged women." Chin J Physiol, 2005 Mar 31;48(1):23-9.

[19] Iwasaki, Y., et al. "Dehydroepiandrosterone-sulfate inhibits nuclear factor-kappaB-dependent transcription in hepatocytes, possibly through antioxidant effect." J Clin Endocrinol Metab, 2004 Jul;89(7):3449-54.

[20] Alhaj, H.A., et al. "Effects of DHEA administration on episodic memory, cortisol and mood in healthy young men: a double-blind, placebo-controlled study." Psychopharmacology (Berl), 2006 Nov;188(4):541-51.

[21] Maninger, N., et al. "Neurobiological and neuropsychiatric effects of dehydroepiandrosterone (DHEA) and DHEA sulfate (DHEAS)." Front Neuroendocrinol, 2009 Jan;30(1):65-91.

[22] Binder, G., et al. "Effects of dehydroepiandrosterone therapy on pubic hair growth and psychological well-being in adolescent girls and young women with central adrenal insufficiency: a double-blind, randomized, placebo-controlled phase III trial." J Clin Endocrinol Metab, 2009 Apr;94(4):1182-90.

[23] Gurnell, E.M., et al. "Long-term DHEA replacement in primary adrenal insufficiency: a randomized, controlled trial." J Clin Endocrinol Metab, 2008 Feb;93(2):400-9.

[24] Artini, P.G., et al. "DHEA supplementation improves follicular microenviroment in poor responder patients." Gynecol Endocrinol, 2012 Sep;28(9):669-73.

[25] Hyman, J.H., et al. "DHEA supplementation may improve IVF outcome in poor responders: a proposed mechanism." Eur J Obstet Gynecol Reprod Biol, 2013 Jan 8. pii: S0301-2115(12)00581-7.

26 Rabijewski, M. and Zgliczyński, W. "Positive effects of DHEA therapy on insulin resistance and lipids in men with angiographically verified coronary heart disease—preliminary study." Endokrynol Pol, 2005 Nov-Dec;56(6):904-10.

27 Yamada, Y., et al. "Changes in serum sex hormone profiles after short-term low-dose administration of dehydroepiandrosterone (DHEA) to young and elderly persons." Endocr J, 2007 Feb;54(1):153-62.

28 Yamada, Y., et al. "Changes in serum sex hormone profiles after short-term low-dose administration of dehydroepiandrosterone (DHEA) to young and elderly persons." Endocr J, 2007 Feb;54(1):153-62.

29 Barrett-Connor, E., et al. "A prospective study of dehydroepiandrosterone sulfate, mortality, and cardiovascular disease." N Engl J Med, 1986 Dec 11;315(24):1519-24.

30 Danforth, K.N., et al. "The association of plasma androgen levels with breast, ovarian and endometrial cancer risk factors among postmenopausal women." Int J Cancer, 2010 Jan 1;126(1):199-207.

31 Tworoger, S.S., et al. "Birthweight and body size throughout life in relation to sex hormones and prolactin concentrations in premenopausal women." Cancer Epidemiol Biomarkers Prev, 2006 Dec;15(12):2494-501.

32 Johnson, M.D., et al. "Uses of DHEA in aging and other disease states." Ageing Res Rev, 2002 Feb;1(1):29-41.

33 Endogenous Hormones and Prostate Cancer Collaborative Group: Roddam, A.W., et al. "Endogenous sex hormones and prostate cancer: a collaborative analysis of 18 prospective studies." J Natl Cancer Inst, 2008 Feb 6;100(3):170-83.

34 Algarté-Génin, M., et al. "Prevention of prostate cancer by androgens: experimental paradox or clinical reality." Eur Urol, 2004 Sep;46(3):285-94.

Chapter 8: Growth Hormone

[1] Rudman, D., et al. "Effects of human growth hormone in men over 60 years old." N Engl J Med, 1990 Jul 5;323(1):1-6.

[2] Powers, M. "Performance-Enhancing Drugs." Principles of Pharmacology for Athletic Trainers, by Houglum, J.E., et al. Thorofare, NJ: SLACK, 2005. 331-32.

[3] Popovic, V., et al. "Hypopituitarism following traumatic brain injury." Growth Horm IGF Res, 2005 Jun;15(3):177-84.

[4] Rohrer, T.R., et al. "Late endocrine sequelae after radiotherapy of pediatric brain tumors are independent of tumor location." J Endocrinol Invest, 2009 Apr;32(4):294-7.

[5] Borson-Chazot, F. and Brue, T. "Pituitary deficiency after brain radiation therapy." Ann Endocrinol (Paris), 2006 Sep;67(4):303-9.

[6] Rudman, D., et al. "Effects of human growth hormone in men over 60 years old." N Engl J Med, 1990 Jul 5;323(1):1-6.

[7] Lanes, R., et al. "Circulating levels of high-sensitivity C-reactive protein and soluble markers of vascular endothelial cell activation in growth hormone-deficient adolescents." Horm Res, 2008;70(4):230-5.

[8] Colao, A. "The GH-IGF-I axis and the cardiovascular system: clinical implications." Clin Endocrinol (Oxf), 2008 Sep;69(3):347-58.

[9] Randeva, H.S., et al. "Growth hormone replacement decreases plasma levels of matrix metalloproteinases (2 and 9) and vascular endothelial growth factor in growth hormone-deficient individuals." Circulation, 2004 May 25;109(20):2405-10.

[10] Kargi, A.Y. and Merriam, G.R. "Testing for growth hormone deficiency in adults: doing without growth hormone-releasing hormone." Curr Opin Endocrinol Diabetes Obes, 2012 Aug;19(4):300-5.

[11] Toogood, A., et al. "Similar clinical features among patients with severe adult growth hormone deficiency diagnosed with insulin tol-

erance test or arginine or glucagon stimulation tests." Endocr Pract, 2012 May-Jun;18(3):325-34.

12 Monson, J.P. "Long-term experience with GH replacement therapy: efficacy and safety." Eur J Endocrinol, 2003 Apr;148 Suppl 2:S9-14.

13 Thomas, J.D. and Monson, J.P. "Adult GH deficiency throughout lifetime." Eur J Endocrinol, 2009 Nov;161 Suppl 1:S97-S106.

14 Tesselaar, K. and Miedema, F. "Growth hormone resurrects adult human thymus during HIV-1 infection." J Clin Invest, 2008 Mar;118(3):844-7.

15 Sleivert, G., et al. "The effects of deer antler velvet extract or powder supplementation on aerobic power, erythropoiesis, and muscular strength and endurance characteristics." Int J Sport Nutr Exerc Metab, 2003 Sep;13(3):251-65.

16 Syrotuik, D.G., et al. "Effect of elk velvet antler supplementation on the hormonal response to acute and chronic exercise in male and female rowers." Int J Sport Nutr Exerc Metab, 2005 Aug;15(4):366-85.

17 Sanders, J.L. and Newman, A.B. "Telomere Length in Epidemiology: A Biomarker of Aging, Age-Related Disease, Both, or Neither?" Epidemiol Rev, 2013 Jan 9. [Epub ahead of print]

18 Mikhelson, V.M. and Gamaley, I.A. "Telomere shortening is a sole mechanism of aging in mammals." Curr Aging Sci, 2012 Dec 1;5(3):203-8.

19 Barbieri, M., et al. "Higher circulating levels of IGF-1 are associated with longer leukocyte telomere length in healthy subjects." Mech Ageing Dev, 2009 Nov-Dec;130(11-12):771-6.

20 Movérare-Skrtic, S., et al. "Serum insulin-like growth factor-I concentration is associated with leukocyte telomere length in a population-based cohort of elderly men." J Clin Endocrinol Metab, 2009 Dec;94(12):5078-84.

Chapter 9: Nutrition

[1] "Size Up Your Sweetener Options."
http://www.forecast.diabetes.org/magazine/food-thought/size-your-sweetener-options

[2] Humphries, P., et al. "Direct and indirect cellular effects of aspartame on the brain." Eur J Clin Nutr, 2008 Apr;62(4):451-62.

[3] Huff, J. and LaDou, J. "Aspartame bioassay findings portend human cancer hazards." Int J Occup Environ Health, 2007 Oct-Dec;13(4):446-8.

[4] Gombos, K., et al. "The effect of aspartame administration on oncogene and suppressor gene expressions." In Vivo, 2007 Jan-Feb;21(1):89-92.

[5] Olney, J.W., et al. "Increasing brain tumor rates: is there a link to aspartame?" J Neuropathol Exp Neurol, 1996 Nov;55(11):1115-23.

[6] Walton, R.G., et al. "Adverse reactions to aspartame: double-blind challenge in patients from a vulnerable population." Biol Psychiatry, 1993 Jul 1-15;34(1-2):13-7.

[7] Van den Eeden, S.K., et al. "Aspartame ingestion and headaches: a randomized crossover trial." Neurology, 1994 Oct;44(10):1787-93.

[8] Roberts, A., et al. "Sucralose metabolism and pharmacokinetics in man." Food Chem Toxicol, 2000;38 Suppl 2:S31-41.

[9] "The Dangers of Chlorine and Issues With Sucralose."
http://articles.mercola.com/sites/articles/archive/2001/06/23/chlorine-part-two.aspx

[10] "Obesity (most recent) by country."
http://www.nationmaster.com/graph/hea_obe-health-obesity

[11] "The prevalence of diabetes has reached epidemic proportions."
http://www.worlddiabetesfoundation.org/composite-35.htm

[12] Walsh, B. "The Real Cost of Cheap Food: America's Food Crisis and How to Fix It." Time, 2009 Aug 31, U.S. Vol. 174 No. 8.

13 Josefson, D. "High insulin levels linked to deaths from breast cancer." BMJ, 2000 Jun 3;320(7248):1496.

14 Kuusisto, J., et al. "Association between features of the insulin resistance syndrome and Alzheimer's disease independently of apolipoprotein E4 phenotype: cross sectional population based study." BMJ, 1997 Oct 25;315(7115):1045-9.

15 Fontbonne, A., et al. "Coronary heart disease mortality risk: plasma insulin level is a more sensitive marker than hypertension or abnormal glucose tolerance in overweight males. The Paris Prospective Study." Int J Obes, 1988;12(6):557-65.

16 Philippou, E., et al. "Preliminary report: the effect of a 6-month dietary glycemic index manipulation in addition to healthy eating advice and weight loss on arterial compliance and 24-hour ambulatory blood pressure in men: a pilot study." Metabolism, 2009 Dec;58(12):1703-8.

17 Simopoulos, A.P. "Omega-3 fatty acids in inflammation and autoimmune diseases." J Am Coll Nutr, 2002 Dec;21(6):495-505.

18 Kim, J., et al. "Fatty fish and fish omega-3 fatty acid intakes decrease the breast cancer risk: a case-control study." BMC Cancer, 2009 Jun 30;9:216.

19 Rupp, H., et al. "Risk stratification by the "EPA+DHA level" and the "EPA/AA ratio" focus on anti-inflammatory and antiarrhythmogenic effects of long-chain omega-3 fatty acids." Herz, 2004 Nov;29(7):673-85.

20 von Schacky, C. "A review of omega-3 ethyl esters for cardiovascular prevention and treatment of increased blood triglyceride levels." Vasc Health Risk Manag, 2006;2(3):251-62.

21 Giovannucci, E., et al. "25-hydroxyvitamin D and risk of myocardial infarction in men: a prospective study." Arch Intern Med, 2008 Jun 9;168(11):1174-80.

[22] Nagpal, S., et al. "Noncalcemic actions of vitamin D receptor ligands." Endocr Rev, 2005 Aug;26(5):662-87.

[23] Freedman, D.M., et al. "Prospective study of serum vitamin D and cancer mortality in the United States." J Natl Cancer Inst, 2007 Nov 7;99(21):1594-602.

[24] Lappe, J.M., et al. "Vitamin D and calcium supplementation reduces cancer risk: results of a randomized trial." Am J Clin Nutr, 2007 Jun;85(6):1586-91.

[25] Sanders, J.L. and Newman, A.B. "Telomere Length in Epidemiology: A Biomarker of Aging, Age-Related Disease, Both, or Neither?" Epidemiol Rev, 2013 Jan 9. [Epub ahead of print]

[26] Mikhelson, V.M. and Gamaley, I.A. "Telomere shortening is a sole mechanism of aging in mammals." Curr Aging Sci, 2012 Dec 1;5(3):203-8.

[27] Xu, Q., et al. "Multivitamin use and telomere length in women." Am J Clin Nutr, 2009 Jun;89(6):1857-63.

[28] Farzaneh-Far, R., et al. "Association of marine omega-3 fatty acid levels with telomeric aging in patients with coronary heart disease." JAMA, 2010 Jan 20;303(3):250-7.

[29] Richards, J.B., et al. "Higher serum vitamin D concentrations are associated with longer leukocyte telomere length in women." Am J Clin Nutr, 2007 Nov;86(5):1420-5.

Chapter 10: Intravenous Nutrition

[1] Milne, G.L., et al. "F2-isoprostanes as markers of oxidative stress in vivo: an overview." Biomarkers, 2005 Nov;10 Suppl 1:S10-23.

[2] Monks, T.J. et al. "Symposium overview: the role of glutathione in neuroprotection and neurotoxicity." Toxicol Sci, 1999 Oct;51(2):161-77.

3 Jana, S. and Mandlekar, S. "Role of phase II drug metabolizing enzymes in cancer chemoprevention." Curr Drug Metab, 2009 Jul;10(6):595-616.

4 Prasad, S.B., et al. "Association of gene polymorphism in detoxification enzymes and urinary 8-OHdG levels in traffic policemen exposed to vehicular exhaust." Inhal Toxicol, 2013 Jan;25(1):1-8.

5 Allen, J. and Bradley, R.D. "Effects of oral glutathione supplementation on systemic oxidative stress biomarkers in human volunteers." J Altern Complement Med, 2011 Sep;17(9):827-33.

6 Chiba, T., et al. "Fas-mediated apoptosis is modulated by intracellular glutathione in human T cells." Eur J Immunol, 1996 May;26(5):1164-9.

7 Berk, M., et al. "The promise of N-acetylcysteine in neuropsychiatry." Trends Pharmacol Sci, 2013 Mar;34(3):167-77.

8 Radtke, K.K., et al. "Interaction of N-acetylcysteine and cysteine in human plasma." J Pharm Sci, 2012 Dec;101(12):4653-9.

9 Martínez-Banaclocha, M.A. "N-acetyl-cysteine in the treatment of Parkinson's disease. What are we waiting for?" Med Hypotheses, 2012 Jul;79(1):8-12.

10 Sekhar, R.V., et al. "Deficient synthesis of glutathione underlies oxidative stress in aging and can be corrected by dietary cysteine and glycine supplementation." Am J Clin Nutr, 2011 Sep;94(3):847-53.

11 Sekhar, R.V., et al. "Glutathione synthesis is diminished in patients with uncontrolled diabetes and restored by dietary supplementation with cysteine and glycine." Diabetes Care, 2011 Jan;34(1):162-7.

12 De Mattia, G., et al. "Influence of reduced glutathione infusion on glucose metabolism in patients with non-insulin-dependent diabetes mellitus." Metabolism, 1998 Aug;47(8):993-7.

[13] Cascinu, S., et al. "Neuroprotective effect of reduced glutathione on oxaliplatin-based chemotherapy in advanced colorectal cancer: a randomized, double-blind, placebo-controlled trial." J Clin Oncol, 2002 Aug 15;20(16):3478-83.

[14] Catarzi, S., et al. "Oxidative state and IL-6 production in intestinal myofibroblasts of Crohn's disease patients." Inflamm Bowel Dis, 2011 Aug;17(8):1674-84.

[15] Guijarro, L.G., et al. "N-acetyl-L-cysteine combined with mesalamine in the treatment of ulcerative colitis: randomized, placebo-controlled pilot study." World J Gastroenterol, 2008 May 14;14(18):2851-7.

[16] De Mattia, G., et al. "Influence of reduced glutathione infusion on glucose metabolism in patients with non-insulin-dependent diabetes mellitus." Metabolism, 1998 Aug;47(8):993-7.

[17] Cascinu, S., et al. "Neuroprotective effect of reduced glutathione on oxaliplatin-based chemotherapy in advanced colorectal cancer: a randomized, double-blind, placebo-controlled trial." J Clin Oncol, 2002 Aug 15;20(16):3478-83.

[18] Sekhar, R.V., et al. "Deficient synthesis of glutathione underlies oxidative stress in aging and can be corrected by dietary cysteine and glycine supplementation." Am J Clin Nutr, 2011 Sep;94(3):847-53.

[19] Exner, R., et al. "Therapeutic potential of glutathione." Wien Klin Wochenschr, 2000 Jul 28;112(14):610-6.

[20] Melhem, A., et al. "Treatment of chronic hepatitis C virus infection via antioxidants: results of a phase I clinical trial." J Clin Gastroenterol, 2005 Sep;39(8):737-42.

[21] Cameron, E. and Pauling, L. "Supplemental ascorbate in the supportive treatment of cancer: Prolongation of survival times in terminal human cancer." Proc Natl Acad Sci U S A, 1976 Oct;73(10):3685-9.

22 Creagan, E.T., et al. "Failure of high-dose vitamin C (ascorbic acid) therapy to benefit patients with advanced cancer. A controlled trial." N Engl J Med, 1979 Sep 27;301(13):687-90.

23 Mayland, C.R., et al. "Vitamin C deficiency in cancer patients." Palliat Med, 2005 Jan;19(1):17-20.

24 Maggini, S., et al. "A combination of high-dose vitamin C plus zinc for the common cold." J Int Med Res, 2012;40(1):28-42.

25 Mikirova, N., et al. "Effect of high-dose intravenous vitamin C on inflammation in cancer patients." J Transl Med, 2012 Sep 11;10:189.

26 Melhem, A., et al. "Treatment of chronic hepatitis C virus infection via antioxidants: results of a phase I clinical trial." J Clin Gastroenterol, 2005 Sep;39(8):737-42.

27 Kodama, M., et al. "Diabetes mellitus is controlled by vitamin C treatment." In Vivo, 1993 Nov-Dec;7(6A):535-42.

28 Murata, A., et al. "Prolongation of survival times of terminal cancer patients by administration of large doses of ascorbate." Int J Vitam Nutr Res Suppl, 1982;23:103-13.

29 Campbell, A., et al. "Reticulum cell sarcoma: two complete 'spontaneous' regressions, in response to high-dose ascorbic acid therapy. A report on subsequent progress." Oncology, 1991;48(6):495-7.

30 Monti, D.A., et al. "Phase I evaluation of intravenous ascorbic acid in combination with gemcitabine and erlotinib in patients with metastatic pancreatic cancer." PLoS One, 2012;7(1):e29794.

31 Cullen, J.J. "Ascorbate induces autophagy in pancreatic cancer." Autophagy, 2010 Apr;6(3):421-2.

32 Vollbracht, C., et al. "Intravenous vitamin C administration improves quality of life in breast cancer patients during chemo-/radiotherapy and aftercare: results of a retrospective, multicentre, epidemiological cohort study in Germany." In Vivo, 2011 Nov-Dec;25(6):983-90.

33 Rees, D.C., et al. "Acute haemolysis induced by high dose ascorbic acid in glucose-6-phosphate dehydrogenase deficiency." BMJ, 1993 Mar 27;306(6881):841-2.

34 Mehta, J.B., et al. "Ascorbic-acid-induced haemolysis in G-6-PD deficiency." Lancet, 1990 Oct 13;336(8720):944.

35 Fox, C., et al. "Magnesium: its proven and potential clinical significance." South Med J, 2001 Dec;94(12):1195-201.

36 McCoy, S. and Baldwin, K. "Pharmacotherapeutic options for the treatment of preeclampsia." Am J Health Syst Pharm, 2009 Feb 15;66(4):337-44.

37 Singh, A.K., et al. "A randomized controlled trial of intravenous magnesium sulphate as an adjunct to standard therapy in acute severe asthma." Iran J Allergy Asthma Immunol, 2008 Dec;7(4):221-9.

38 Mauskop, A., et al. "Intravenous magnesium sulfate rapidly alleviates headaches of various types." Headache, 1996 Mar;36(3):154-60.

39 Bayir, A., et al. "Magnesium sulfate in emergency department patients with hypertension." Biol Trace Elem Res, 2009 Apr;128(1):38-44.

40 Stremmel, W., et al. "Retarded release phosphatidylcholine benefits patients with chronic active ulcerative colitis." Gut, 2005 Jul;54(7):966-71.

41 Hayashi, H., et al. "Beneficial effect of salmon roe phosphatidylcholine in chronic liver disease." Curr Med Res Opin, 1999;15(3):177-84.

42 Schaefer, E.J., et al. "Plasma phosphatidylcholine docosahexaenoic acid content and risk of dementia and Alzheimer disease: the Framingham Heart Study." Arch Neurol, 2006 Nov;63(11):1545-50.

43 Kuo, H.W., et al. "Urinary 8-hydroxy-2'-deoxyguanosine (8-OHdG) and genetic polymorphisms in breast cancer patients." Mutat Res, 2007 Jul 10;631(1):62-8.

Chapter 11: Detoxification

1 Roy, J.R., et al. "Estrogen-like endocrine disrupting chemicals affecting puberty in humans—a review." Med Sci Monit, 2009 Jun;15(6):RA137-45.

2 Androutsopoulos, V.P., et al. "Cytochrome P450 CYP1A1: wider roles in cancer progression and prevention." BMC Cancer, 2009 Jun 16;9:187.

3 Rupp, H., et al. "Risk stratification by the "EPA+DHA level" and the "EPA/AA ratio" focus on anti-inflammatory and antiarrhythmogenic effects of long-chain omega-3 fatty acids." Herz, 2004 Nov;29(7):673-85.

4 Trinh, K.J., et al. "Induction of the phase II detoxification pathway suppresses neuron loss in Drosophila models of Parkinson's disease." Neurosci, 2008 Jan 9;28(2):465-72.

5 Bagga, D., et al. "Effects of a very low fat, high fiber diet on serum hormones and menstrual function. Implications for breast cancer prevention." Cancer, 1995 Dec 15;76(12):2491-6.

6 Forman, M.R. "Changes in dietary fat and fiber and serum hormone concentrations: nutritional strategies for breast cancer prevention over the life course." J Nutr, 2007 Jan;137(1 Suppl):170S-174S.

7 Adlercreutz, H., et al. "Estrogen metabolism and excretion in Oriental and Caucasian women." J Natl Cancer Inst, 1994 Jul 20;86(14):1076-82.

8 Im, A., et al. "Urinary estrogen metabolites in women at high risk for breast cancer." Carcinogenesis, 2009 Sep;30(9):1532-5.

9 Kabat, G.C., et al. "Estrogen metabolism and breast cancer." Epidemiology, 2006 Jan;17(1):80-8.

10 Massart, F., et al. "How do environmental estrogen disruptors induce precocious puberty?" Minerva Pediatr, 2006 Jun;58(3):247-54.

11 Roy, J.R., et al. "Estrogen-like endocrine disrupting chemicals affecting puberty in humans—a review." Med Sci Monit, 2009 Jun;15(6):RA137-45.

12 Alonso-Magdalena, P., et al. "The estrogenic effect of bisphenol A disrupts pancreatic beta-cell function in vivo and induces insulin resistance." Environ Health Perspect, 2006 Jan;114(1):106-12.

13 "Cigarette Smoking."
http://www.cancer.org/docroot/PED/content/PED_10_2X_Cigarette_Smoking.asp?sitearea=PED

14 Fagerberg, B., et al. "C-reactive protein and tumor necrosis factor-alpha in relation to insulin-mediated glucose uptake, smoking and atherosclerosis." Scand J Clin Lab Invest, 2008 Feb 18:1-8.

15 Cheng, S.E., et al. "Cigarette smoke extract induces cytosolic phospholipase A2 expression via NADPH oxidase, MAPKs, AP-1, and NF-kappaB in human tracheal smooth muscle cells." Free Radic Biol Med, 2009 Apr 1;46(7):948-60.

16 Halvorsen, B., et al. "Effect of smoking cessation on markers of inflammation and endothelial cell activation among individuals with high risk for cardiovascular disease." Scand J Clin Lab Invest, 2007;67(6):604-11.

17 Valavanidis, A., et al. "8-hydroxy-2'-deoxyguanosine (8-OHdG): A critical biomarker of oxidative stress and carcinogenesis." J Environ Sci Health C Environ Carcinog Ecotoxicol Rev, 2009 Apr;27(2):120-39.

18 Androutsopoulos, V.P., et al. "Cytochrome P450 CYP1A1: wider roles in cancer progression and prevention." BMC Cancer, 2009 Jun 16;9:187.

19 Trinh, K., et al. "Induction of the phase II detoxification pathway suppresses neuron loss in Drosophila models of Parkinson's disease." J Neurosci, 2008 Jan 9;28(2):465-72.

20 Vassalle, C., et al. "Evidence for enhanced 8-isoprostane plasma levels, as index of oxidative stress in vivo, in patients with coronary artery disease." Artery Dis, 2003 May;14(3):213-8.

21 Chen, C.M., et al. "Increased oxidative damage in peripheral blood correlates with severity of Parkinson's disease." Neurobiol Dis, 2009 Mar;33(3):429-35.

22 Du, Y., et al. "Oxidative damage to the promoter region of SQSTM1/p62 is common to neurodegenerative disease." Neurobiol Dis, 2009 Aug;35(2):302-10.

23 Abder-Rahman, H.A. and Nusair, S. "8-Hydroxy-2'-deoxyguanosine (8-OHdG) as a short-term predictor of regional and occupational health problems." J UOEH, 2007 Sep 1;29(3):247-58.

24 Nishikawa, T., et al. "Evaluation of urinary 8-hydroxydeoxy-guanosine as a novel biomarker of macrovascular complications in type 2 diabetes." Diabetes Care, 2003 May;26(5):1507-12.

Chapter 12: Exercise

1 Kasapis, C. and Thompson, P.D. "The effects of physical activity on serum C-reactive protein and inflammatory markers: a systematic review." J Am Coll Cardiol, 2005 May 17;45(10):1563-9.

Chapter 13: Sleep

1 Smits, M.G., et al. "Melatonin improves health status and sleep in children with idiopathic chronic sleep-onset insomnia: a random-ized, placebo-controlled trial." J Am Acad Child Adolesc Psychiatry, 2003 Nov;42(11):1286-93.

2 Hoebert, M., et al. "Long-term follow-up of melatonin treatment in children with ADHD and chronic sleep onset insomnia." J Pineal Res, 2009 Aug;47(1):1-7.

3 Ivanenko, A., et al. "Melatonin in children and adolescents with insomnia: a retrospective study." Clin Pediatr (Phila), 2003
   Jan-Feb;42(1):51-8.

4 Andréen, L., et al. "Sex steroid induced negative mood may be explained by the paradoxical effect mediated by GABAA modulators."
   Psychoneuroendocrinology, 2009 Sep;34(8):1121-32.

5 Maes, M. "The cytokine hypothesis of depression: inflammation,
   oxidative & nitrosative stress (IO&NS) and leaky gut as new targets
   for adjunctive treatments in depression." Neuro Endocrinol Lett,
   2008 Jun;29(3):287-91.

6 Maes, M., et al. "The inflammatory & neurodegenerative (I&ND)
   hypothesis of depression: leads for future research and new drug
   developments in depression." Metab Brain Dis, 2009
   Mar;24(1):27-53.

7 Miller, M.A., et al. "Gender differences in the cross-sectional relationships between sleep duration and markers of inflammation:
   Whitehall II study." Sleep, 2009 Jul 1;32(7):857-64.

8 Simpson, N. and Dinges, D.F. "Sleep and inflammation." Nutr Rev,
   2007 Dec;65(12 Pt 2):S244-52.

9 "Night-shift work linked to cancer."
   http://www.usatoday.com/news/health/2007-11-29-night-shift-can
   cer_N.htm

10 Maes, M. "The cytokine hypothesis of depression: inflammation,
    oxidative & nitrosative stress (IO&NS) and leaky gut as new targets
    for adjunctive treatments in depression." Neuro Endocrinol Lett,
    2008 Jun;29(3):287-91.

11 Maes, M., et al. "The inflammatory & neurodegenerative (I&ND)
    hypothesis of depression: leads for future research and new drug
    developments in depression." Metab Brain Dis, 2009
    Mar;24(1):27-53.

Chapter 14: Laughter

[1] Berk L.S., et al. "Neuroendocrine and stress hormone changes during mirthful laughter." Am J Med Sci, 1989 Dec;298(6):390-6.

Chapter 15: Energy Production

[1] Ghirlanda, G., et al. "Evidence of plasma CoQ10-lowering effect by HMG-CoA reductase inhibitors: a double-blind, placebo-controlled study." J Clin Pharmacol, 1993 Mar;33(3):226-9.

[2] Marcoff, L. and Thompson, P.D. "The role of coenzyme Q10 in statin-associated myopathy: a systematic review." J Am Coll Cardiol, 2007 Jun 12;49(23):2231-7.

[3] Kishi, T., et al. "Bioenergetics in clinical medicine XV. Inhibition of coenzyme Q10-enzymes by clinically used adrenergic blockers of beta-receptors." Res Commun Chem Pathol Pharmacol, 1977 May;17(1):157-64.

[4] Kishi, H., et al. "Bioenergetics in clinical medicine. III. Inhibition of coenzyme Q10-enzymes by clinically used anti-hypertensive drugs." Res Commun Chem Pathol Pharmacol, 1975 Nov;12(3):533-40.

[5] Tonda, M.E. and Hart, L.L. "N,N dimethylglycine and L-carnitine as performance enhancers in athletes." Ann Pharmacother, 1992 Jul-Aug;26(7-8):935-7.

Appendix: Inflammation

[1] Roubenoff, R., et al. "Cytokines, insulin-like growth factor-1, sarcopenia, and mortality in very old community-dwelling men and women: the Framingham Heart Study." Am J Med, 2003 Oct 15;115(6):429-35.

[2] Sullivan, D.H., et al. "Association between inflammation-associated cytokines, serum albumins, and mortality in the elderly." J Am Med Dir Assoc, 2007 Sep;8(7):458-63.

[3] Tsimberidou, A.M., et al. "The prognostic significance of cytokine levels in newly diagnosed acute myeloid leukemia and high-risk myelodysplastic syndromes." Cancer, 2008 Oct 1;113(7):1605-13.

[4] Miettinen, K.H., et al. "Prognostic role of pro- and anti-inflammatory cytokines and their polymorphisms in acute decompensated heart failure." Eur J Heart Fail, 2008 Apr;10(4):396-403.

INDEX

Charts

Numerical

A

F

food allergy— 32

Food and Drug Administration—See FDA.

food intolerance—See delayed food sensitivity.

formaldehyde— 140-141, 176

formic acid— 140-141

Framingham Heart Study— 232

free radical(s)— 15, 81, 84, 97, 113, 135, 158, 174, 178-179, 181, 185, 218, 222

G

GABA (gamma-aminobutyric acid)— 47, 197, 201

gamma-aminobutyric acid—See GABA.

gamma-tocotrienol— 82

Genova Diagnostics®— 82, 104, 233

ghrelin— 125

glucagon— 132

gluten— 20, 23, 25-26, 31

glutathione— 82, 150, 155, 157-160, 163-164, 170-172, 174, 178, 181, 219, 222

glycemic diet— 147-148, 151

Graves' disease— 56

growth hormone— 7, 9, 43, 125-129, 131-137, 152, 201, 204-205, 207, 210, 214, 220-221

gut— 6, 10, 17, 19-36, 46, 50, 199-201, 203, 209, 215-216, 220, 225, 227-228

H

Hashimoto's thyroiditis— 54-55

HCG (human chorionic gonadotropin)— 6, 110, 114

HGH (human growth hormone)— 126, 131-134, 136, 204, 207

headache(s)— 33, 35, 44, 69, 71, 89, 97, 132, 140, 165, 198, 212

R

reproductive— 2, 44, 87

resveratrol— 82

rhodiola rosea— 48, 210

Rossouw, Jacques, Dr.— 67

Rudman, Daniel, Dr.— 131

S

saliva— 26, 33, 40, 45, 50, 98, 117, 123, 196, 204, 210, 215

saliva glands— 40

seizure(s)— 44, 57, 65, 140

selective serotonin reuptake inhibitor (SSRI)— 198

selenium— 55, 58, 63

Selye, Hans, Dr.— 40, 42

serotonin— 11, 198-201

sex hormone binding globulin (SHBG)— 40

SHBG—See sex hormone binding globulin.

short stature— 131

skin— 3, 20, 29, 31, 33, 41, 44, 54, 65, 70, 72, 118, 126, 131, 137, 148, 164, 171, 178, 214, 219

sleep— 3-5, 10-11, 38, 41-43, 45, 47-48, 50, 89-90, 93, 96, 98, 106, 125, 134-136, 160, 186, 195-201, 209-210, 212, 215, 219-220, 223, 225, 227

sinusitis— 33

sleep apnea— 3, 198, 201, 210

smoking— 13, 70, 176, 180, 187, 220, 223, 231

somatostatin— 126

SSRI— See selective serotonin reuptake inhibitor.

steroid(s)— 19-22, 28, 55, 75, 117, 174, 216

strength training— 188, 191, 194

W

X

Y

BIOGRAPHY AND
ADDITIONAL READING

Edwin N. Lee is a medical doctor, author and spokesperson who—thanks in part to his groundbreaking insight in his field, and his many significant presentations at major medical conferences around the world—is a respected proponent and authority on hormonal balance and wellness, and a renowned leader in defining the future of regenerative and functional medicine.

He is board certified in Internal Medicine, Endocrinology, Diabetes and Metabolism, and has completed special courses in Regenerative and Functional Medicine. And, he is the assistant professor of Internal Medicine at the University of Central Florida College of Medicine.

Dr. Lee founded the Institute for Hormonal Balance in 2008. His driving purpose for opening the Institute was being able to focus on prevention of diseases, rather than just treating the impact of diseases—that in many cases could have been prevented.

Hormonal balance, with bioidentical or natural hormones, is the cornerstone for keeping the body and mind healthy. The Institute for Hormonal Balance has a holistic approach to integrating the best of western and eastern medicine, thereby improving the mind, body and soul so that one can heal naturally.

Dr. Lee graduated from the Medical College of Pennsylvania, completed three years of Internal Medicine residency and then completed two fellowships—in Endocrinology and Metabolism, and in Critical Care Medicine—at the University of Pittsburgh. He also served as the

Team Endocrinologist for the Cleveland Indians during their spring training in Florida.

In addition to writing his books, *Feel Good Look Younger: Reversing Tiredness Through Hormonal Balance* and *Your Best Investment: Secrets to a Healthy Body and Mind*, Dr. Lee has written many articles on internal medicine and endocrinology.

He was also an author in the fourth edition of *Textbook of Critical Care* in the chapter entitled, Neuroendocrine Immunology and the Role of Neuroendocrine Hormones in the Critically Ill Patient.

Dr. Lee is an active member of the Age Management Medicine Group, the American Academy of Anti-Aging and the American Association of Clinical Endocrinology.

He truly enjoys helping his patients achieve better health, and is known for practicing what he preaches. Dr. Lee has completed several marathons and triathlons, such as the Great Floridian Triathlon (Ironman distance).

Learn the Secrets to a Healthy Heart

Dr. Lee's *Your Amazing Heart* (the kids book that's not just for kids) is first in a series on children's health and nutrition, and has received a Moonbeam Children's Book Award. It is available in print and e-book from Amazon and iTunes.

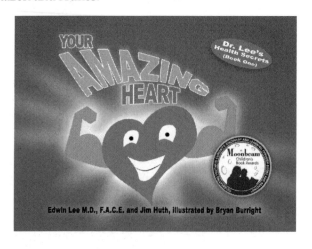

For Additional Reading

Also, be sure to read Dr. Lee's *Your Best Investment: Secrets to a Healthy Body and Mind,* available in print and e-book from Amazon and dredwinlee.com. Written by Dr. Lee to squarely address today's issues of proper nutrition—and to provide his unique, two-phase diet approach—the book has proven to be an easy-to-follow and valuable resource that physicians are now recommending to their patients for straightforward answers on nutrition and preventive medicine.

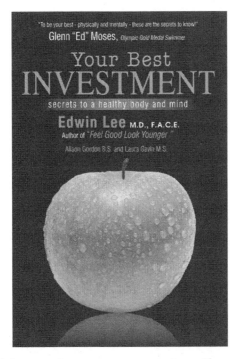

"Dr. Lee will forever change your perception of how simple applications of optimal nutrition can transform your life. This is the diet book that you definitely need to embrace and fully understand."

— Mark Houston MD, MS, FACP, FAHA
Associate Clinical Professor of Medicine
Vanderbilt University Medical School
Director Hypertension Institute
Saint Thomas Medical Group, Nashville, Tennessee
Author of *What Your Doctor May Not Tell You About Hypertension*

"Dr. Lee's well-researched, *Your Best Investment,* as well as his other book, *Feel Good Look Younger,* provide valuable knowledge that can be easily comprehended and applied by all those who share a passion for life."

— Sanjay Banerji, M.D.,
Clinical Professor UCLA Department of Neurology
Consultant Neurologist at Good Samaritan Hospital and
Saint Vincent's Medical Center, Los Angeles, California

"In his book, *Your Best Investment,* Dr. Lee gives you the knowledge and the resources you need to develop a healthy body and mind. Thank you, Dr. Lee!"

— Douglas C. Hall, M.D.
Board Certified in Obstetrics and Gynecology
Functional Medicine, Ocala, Florida

"I have great respect for Dr. Edwin Lee and his work on achieving optimal health through optimal nutrition."

— Dr. Larry Merkle
Clinical Associate Professor of Medicine
Penn State University College of Medicine
Chief Endocrinologist
Lehigh Valley Hospital, Allentown, Pennsylvania